Thank you to absolutely everyone who's been part of my journey in whatever way, however big or small.

Everything happened exactly how it had to be!

First published in 2026 by Intellectual Perspective Press

To find out more about our authors and books visit:

www.intellectualperspective.com

The Drunk Gambler
with Erectile Dysfunction
Searching for Something More

TOM JENKINS

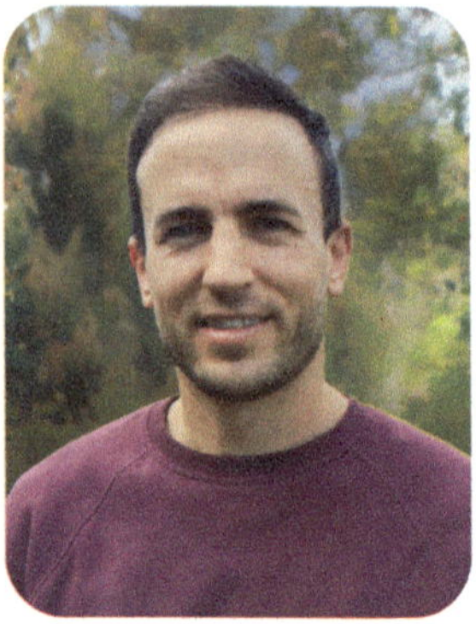

Tom Jenkins is a Brit living in Colombia trying to work out his path in life and what the hell he's doing here.

He's experimented with most things, taking many of them to extremes – from alcohol to drugs, gambling to cults, meditation to psychedelics, and a load of other stuff in the middle.

He's lived a sexual journey of disaster, confusion and complete embarrassment that has slowly evolved into something majestic, featuring many setbacks and a little heartbreak along the way too.

At the age of thirty-six he's put his heart into this book with no detail held back – however shameful, embarrassing or magical some of his stories may be.

He shares what he's learned along the way. Maybe you'll learn something from it; maybe you won't. He's clear that we all have different paths after all, but he does thoroughly hope you enjoy the read.

Thoughts About The Author and The Drunk Gambler with Erectile Dysfunction

'The most transparent book I've ever read about modern struggles with masculinity. Tom openly discusses themes that no one is talking about but lots of men are going through'

- Michael Hanson

'On the surface Tom appears perfectly ordinary. Fortunately, that is not the case'

- Joseph Sandall

'Few people show loyalty, integrity, and generosity as consistently as Tom does, all while keeping his untethered joy for life. I wish everyone could have a friend like him'

- Bennet Hütter

'Tom is completely bonkers. A rollercoaster read where you'll learn how not to make the mistakes he has'

- Tom Lovelace

'Contrary to much that's been written, Tom is one of the most principled and trustworthy men I know'

- Pierre-Yves Beauchemin

Why?

I was never meant to be a guru.

The first time I got drunk was the day I knew I wanted to stop. Eleven years later – after a drink-driving disaster, a twenty-four-hour ban from my local town, being physically assaulted in the back room of a Guildford nightclub by two bouncers, an arrest in New Zealand, delving into cocaine in the largest favela in Rio de Janeiro, becoming mildly insane from edibles in a hippie community in Australia, stealing the credit card machine from a local kebab shop, and a whole lot more – and I finally stopped.

The first time I gambled, I loved it. I bet on Arsenal to beat Southampton 3–1 on a cold night at Highbury on 4 December 1996, and it came through. Fifteen years later, having lost thousands on anything from virtual blackjack to Lithuanian basketball, I quit.

And now, twenty-nine years on from that bet, I'm still searching for more – my path, the way, contentment, purpose or whatever you want to call it. Truth be told, I don't think we ever stop looking for something more.

I could never lead a normal life, never sustain the commuter train, the white picket fence, the Matrix.

In telling my story, I'm aware that many people are getting pissed off with all the spiritual gurus, experts and influencers telling them how to live their lives. So, as you're maybe already pissed off with them, I figured I'd join in and do the same thing too.

Although as the drunk gambler with erectile dysfunction, I hope I'm a little more relatable. Sure, many of these gurus have a backstory, like living on their friend's couch with only a few dollars in their pocket. But those stories rarely include the depths of spiritual and emotional hell, complete sexual failure and embarrassment, or pissing yourself in the corner of a stairwell in a tower block in a city you don't know... with no idea how you got there.

These days, thanks to the experiences I've lived, I've reached a level of contentment, ease, confidence, passion and vision that I never thought possible. All mixed in with a healthy dose of anxiety and confusion, which I'm still working my way through.

I know I'm lucky. Not everyone is born into a situation, a country and a position where they can live all the experiences I have, make the mistakes I have, fall back on support when they mess up, and keep moving forwards. I'm very aware of this. I was born in the UK, in a very nice part of the country, into a wealthy family.

However, there are many other lucky people who could choose a different path but don't. And there are many less fortunate people who could make better decisions that would cost nothing and even save them time and money, but don't.

It's the case for so many people.

People who keep drinking more than they want to. People who never try to find their purpose, stuck inside the system, doing the same commute to a job that was never their dream or passion. People who can't stop worrying about what other people think, locked in a cycle of anxiety and self-doubt, who never feel truly at home in their own body. People who keep staring at porn rather than getting out there and trying to find a real connection.

To me, this is sad. I know; I've lived all of it. To many people who are following that path now, I'm mad – and that's fine. We all live the path that we see as best for us.

I used to really care what people thought of me. Now, for the most part, I don't give a fuck.

So why am I sharing my stories and my journey here?

Firstly, I couldn't sleep one night, so I thought I'd start writing a book.

Secondly, I hope that if you're searching for your meaning or your spiritual path, you might relate to my journey, find some help in it, let go of some confusions, and move closer to where you want to be. You might be taking some vices slightly too far; you might have fucked up in similar ways to me; or you might be constantly worrying about what other people think and yearning for just a little inner tranquillity.

Thirdly, confusion about sexuality, erectile dysfunction, debilitating sexual embarrassment, addiction to porn, and visiting prostitutes are still subjects that people don't truly share or talk about, even though so many of us are going through these struggles. This leaves many people feeling confusion, shame or fear when it comes to sex and sexuality. If that's you, this book might show you that you're not alone: so many of the things you're struggling with, I've been through too – and so are many other people at this very moment. If that's *not* you, I think you'll still enjoy the stories. After all, my first time could have hardly gone worse.

Lastly, I want to share a story that comes from the brutal and simple truth, not from the lofty position of a spiritual oracle.

In all this, I know that no single path works for everyone. The best path I've found – to make a load of mistakes, do a load of things right, push my limits, learn, grow, move forward, and share and understand that what's right for me – may not be what's right for you.

Through stories, I hope we can connect, I hope you'll enjoy the read, and I hope you'll learn something from it – just as I'm sure that if you wrote a book, I'd learn something from you.

* * * * *

All the stories in this book are true. However, many of the names and some minor details have been changed to protect the identities of other people involved.

Enjoy!

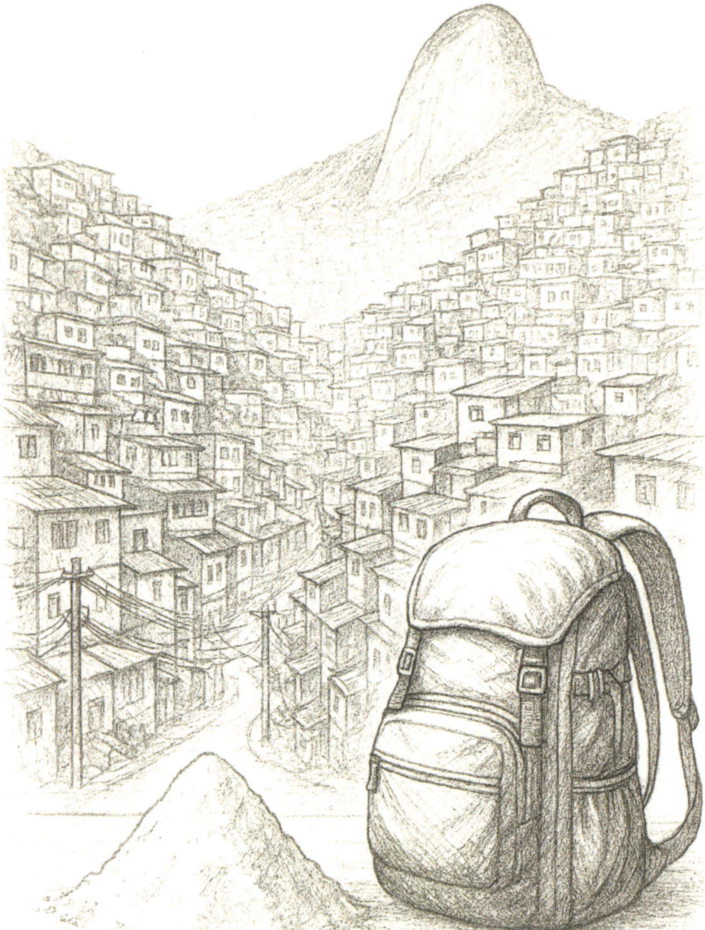

1. Cocaine and Robbery: The Search Begins

It was at Nairobi airport in Kenya that the first monumental shift in my life took place.

It was the summer of 2010, between my second and third year of university. I was twenty one. I'd gone to Nottingham to study geography. Not because I had any passion for geography, saw any real use in it, or even saw any use in going to university – simply because I didn't know what else to do. That's what my brother had done, and I figured, 'Why not follow?'

After all, I had no passion, energy or guiding light at this time to conceive of doing anything else. If I could go back now, I'd drop out of university, not waste any more time there, and do something different with my life. But that's easy for me to say now.

At university I did nothing but drink and waste my time. To describe my first two years as anything but wasted time would be a lie. Sure, I ended up with a half-decent grade, but it only took me one week to learn how to study, remember useless information and pass an exam.

To tell of all the absurd things I did during this time and my teenage years before could go on for seven chapters, but here are two that took place in my first year at university.

One Thursday, I went with Tim, a good friend from Manchester, to Cheltenham horse racing. The night before, I'd been thrown out of one of Nottingham's nightclubs. At the time, it was called Isis – I guess this was before the other notorious group with the same name had become famous.

I don't remember why I was thrown out, but that happened a lot in those days.

After getting a train to Cheltenham, I met Tim and we went to the races. We lost money on every race, and the only way to get over that was to go out and continue drinking. Tim ended the night in a strip club; I was too drunk to be allowed in. I can't really remember any of it.

We were meant to be staying at a friend of Tim's. I didn't know the person, where their house was, or how to get there. Even if I did, I was so drunk, I wouldn't have ended up there anyway.

The night passed, and in the morning, I was woken up in the stairwell of one of the University of Gloucestershire's halls of residence. I had never been to that university, had no idea where it was, and God knows how I'd ended up there.

I'd pissed in the corner of the stairwell right next to the concrete on which I was sleeping, and a little urine had been soaked up by my jeans and jumper. The perfect way to start the day!

The student who found me outside his living quarters wasn't happy. He kicked me out, insisting on searching me before I left to ensure I hadn't stolen anything. However, it seemed that someone had stolen from *me*. Once outside, I realised I had no wallet, no phone, no keys – just the clothes I was wearing.

To be fair, looking back, it's more likely that I'd lost everything through pure drunken stupidity than from theft.

I found a payphone. (This was back in the day when every payphone wasn't a smashed-up urinal.) I called Tim, reversing the charges.* Luckily, he answered. We agreed to meet in the McDonald's in Cheltenham city centre, where we'd eaten the day before. In those days, McDonald's was a regular dining experience and meeting point for me.

I still had no idea where I was. After asking around, I found out that the city centre was forty-five minutes' walk in the freezing cold. We eventually met there. Tim treated me to some McNuggets and then leant me money to get back to Nottingham.

A few months later, I was pulled over by the police. Coincidentally, I'd been thrown out of the same club, Isis, that night too.

I'd gone with a friend, Jeff. We hadn't been planning to go out that night, but at the last minute we decided we would. Isis was an out-of-town club in a shopping complex,

---

* A reverse-charge call is when you call a number and divert the costs of the call to the other person – if they accept. This was also in the days when we remembered people's phone numbers.

so we decided to drive there. We got there at ten o'clock, drank a bottle of Sainsbury's Basics vodka in the car park, then went in. I said with 100% certainty that I'd leave the car there and pick it up the next day: I would never drink and drive.

As the detectives among you have probably guessed, that didn't happen.

When you're smashed off your face, your decision making can become questionable. Another friend, Max, had been thrown out with me. What to do? Get a £5 taxi or drive home? It was only five minutes away. Why not?

I had the perfect solution: I knew I was drunk, so I'd drive super-slow, at five miles an hour. That way, nothing could go wrong... It was also dark, and the streets were lit, so I forgot to turn my lights on.

Two minutes later, blue lights were flashing behind me. I couldn't help wondering how they knew I was drink-driving.

I pulled over, got out of the car, put my hands up and said, 'You've got me, I'm drink-driving.' What was the point in trying to deny it? I was smashed. They pulled out the breathalyser. I told them there really was no need, I was well over the limit; but still, it was procedure.

On the positive side, the police report said something along the lines of me being one of the politest and most apologetic drink-drivers they'd ever arrested if I remember correctly.

At least I'd learned good manners from my childhood and adolescence.

They took me back to Nottingham police station and put me in a cell. I threw up in the metal toilet, passed out, and was woken by the arrival of prison breakfast in bed: sausage and baked beans in a tin-foil tray.

I wasn't really feeling in the mood for breakfast.

When I was let out shortly afterwards, I had to walk back to the university feeling like a true piece of shit.

A month later, I went to court with my dad, pleaded guilty, made my apologies, and got a hefty fine and a two-year driving ban. All wholly deserved, I might add, and I was genuinely sorry. The level I was over the limit by put me in the bracket to be handed community service, but luckily, I escaped that. I also had to attend a drink-driving course, where I met a load of other very messed-up characters completely lost in society – one insisting that he shouldn't be there despite the fact that he said he had tried to attack two cops.

Now let's get back to Nairobi airport.

Three days before that, I'd been in Brazil with Tim.

We'd been to the favela** of Rocinha in Rio de Janeiro. Rocinha is South America's biggest favela, and it has one of the most beautiful views of the Atlantic Ocean you'll ever see. In Rio and in many other parts of South

** A Brazilian word roughly meaning shanty town.

America, the favelas have the most incredible views, because they're built on the hillsides. The flipside is that these zones are usually underdeveloped because they're geographically unstable.

The favelas of Brazil are also where you can meet some amazing communities of incredible people doing their best to get by and help one another. The story I'm going to tell here involves a small minority of these areas, where the social problems are made worse by, well, people like me.

We didn't go to Rocinha with an organised tour guide. We went with a guy who knew a guy from there, Ricardo, who knew the backstreets.

We met some gang members, held their machine guns, and saw a sizeable amount of cocaine. The photos of us with the guns were even on Facebook at one point; thankfully, they've disappeared now. We had to leave a little extra cash for this 'privilege', which was no doubt used to finance that way of life and the drug wars that are still going on today.

Afterwards, we went to a local bar down a side street. I was twenty years old, and cocaine was one of the few things I'd never tried. So, I thought, 'When better to try it than in the backstreets of a Brazilian favela ravaged by past violence and conflict, partly due to the fight for control of cocaine?'

I loved it! I was full of life, full of energy, full of confidence to talk shit about whatever I wanted. I knew it was all bullshit that would wear off to a horrible low after a while, but as a clueless twenty-year-old lost in the moment, who cared? Except we were in the middle of the favela, a long way from our hostel, and it probably wasn't a good place to be high off my face.

As may be expected, after the initial sensation wore off, I only wanted more. We were with a few people who had more sense than Tim and I did, and they wisely decided it was time to find our way back to the main street and take a taxi back to our hostel – Mellow Yellow, next to the Cardeal Arcoverde Metro station in Copacabana. Fortunately, we listened and followed – extra gear in pocket, of course.

The journey back to the hostel went surprisingly smoothly, given where we were, but the party only continued there. I couldn't get enough of the cocaine. Tim tried to make me stop, locking me out of the toilet while he indulged. But I climbed over the top of the cubicle. I wanted more! And I was going to get more! He gave in and left me a little.

I ditched the traditional bank note and ground my face onto the toilet seat, snorting up every last bit I could before coming out looking like a snowman. Tim dusted my face and body off, and we went back out to the bar.

For some inexplicable and truly dickheadish reason, a little after that, I went to our hostel dormitory, threw a load of load of things around – some mine, some not. I was like a messed-up rock-star with none of the glamour and all of the shame. Needless to say, I pissed a whole load of people off.

Half of the rest of what happened, I can't remember. I couldn't walk properly the next day because my right foot was killing me. It was completely swollen.

Thankfully, we were leaving that day. We also hadn't paid our bill. This was the perfect excuse to keep our heads low, sneak out of the hostel, do a runner without paying, and take a taxi to the airport.

Another truly dickheadish move.

When you add the comedown from the coke, alcohol, awful behaviour and so much more from the previous two weeks to a twelve-hour overnight flight back to London before then heading to Nairobi shortly after, this really was rock bottom.

Back to Nairobi airport. I was off to Malawi to volunteer with a microloan charity for three weeks. Yes, that's right: the white person who had done all the things I've confessed in this chapter was off to support black people in poverty in Africa.

I truly felt like shit. How could I not? I deserved to feel like shit.

There I was, sitting outside a tiny bookstore in the airport. I looked up, and my eyes rested on a self-help book. The first I'd ever seen.

It was Robin Sharma's *Life Lessons from a Monk Who Sold His Ferrari*.

It called me in; I bought it and instantly began reading it. And in that moment, it felt like I had finally found a place of hope, some refuge. A guide. My bible, if you must!

From what I remember, it was a list of one hundred steps that could help you change your life. I really tried to follow them. Help people, live in the present, exercise, eat well. It's often those basic and obvious things that we forget In our darkest times that we first have to get back to.

To clarify, I was an extreme binge-drinker, not an alcoholic. I could happily go without drinking all week or all month if I stayed at home, but nearly every time I went out, I'd end up at the stage of blackout or worse.

The people I spent time with at this point were similar to me in their drinking habits and life choices, though perhaps to a less extreme level. I did my best to hide much of it from my parents, lying to them about many things, but I'm sure deep down they felt something was wrong and they were worried.

Mostly, though, I got by. The majority of the time I was a nice, kind, timid kid. But I lacked a huge amount of self-confidence and a healthy dose of self-control when under the influence.

My behaviour around drink and drugs was an attempt to mask the complete lack of self-worth that I'd developed from childhood and through adolescence. It never worked – it only made things worse – but at least for a few hours, there was some escape. When I stayed at home, I was so far inside my tiny comfort zone that I was protected, but that wasn't what I wanted to do. Staying in, I was unbelievably lonely. This is a conundrum faced by so many today.

All this made my three weeks in Africa a good time to make a change and try something new. I wouldn't be drinking or doing anything else – just trying to help (or perhaps better put, not get in the way too much). From a personal point of view, it was an amazing experience.

I stayed with a local guy, Chippie, and his family in a mud house. I followed him around at the charity, I met a lot of locals (who loved meeting a foreigner), and the charity really did do some great work.

It felt good. I felt better. I realised that you can't rub out the mistakes of the past; they're what make you who you are today. That was my big lesson from this time. I'd had good moments from the past too, but it was the bad ones that had stuck.

Over the next few years, I read several other self-help books as the industry boomed. They certainly helped me and gave me a little light that I was searching for at times.

But even though each book I read gave me a little boost, none of them took me to the root of the problem or helped me find the real answers I was looking for. And I often ended up in a cycle of reading book after book, repeating bullshit positivity after bullshit positivity, and forgetting half the 'lessons' I learned a few days on, often ending up with more questions than answers.

That said, I'll be forever grateful for Sharma's book, because in my ultimate low it gave me a way forward, with some practical advice I could use to dig myself out of the hole I'd created for myself. Mixed with the motivation that I never wanted to go back to the state I'd just been in, it worked: from here onwards, I began to take the first steps towards overcoming the gremlins deep inside me. There were many to overcome, and many more mistakes to make – but from this point, the will to overcome them was there.

To make some amends for my behaviour in Brazil, I returned to Rio five years later in a much better state and went back to the hostel to admit what I'd done and pay what I owed. I doubted they'd even remember me or have the information, but I'd calculated the rough amount and fully intended to pay it back.

When I arrived at the door, the hostel had closed down. This made me feel bad. Was I to blame? Perhaps to a small degree.

I instead donated the money to the Ayrton Senna Foundation. Senna is a hero of mine as he is for many Brazilians, and the foundation is a great charity offering great opportunities for the youth of Brazil. With my donation, I explained exactly what I'd done and why I was donating that amount.

Did it cancel out the past? No. But it was the closest thing I felt I could do to make amends.

Reflection #1: The Past Is in the Past

The lesson here is the old cliché: the past is in the past.

Sure, I'd brought drugs into the hostel, gone out of control and then did a runner without paying my bill...

I'll hold my hands up: that's not good in anyone's book, especially my own. But until someone invents a time machine, I can't change that. And sitting in a pile of shit feeling awful about it only made things worse.

There came a point where I had a choice to make: do I stay there repeating the same shit again and again, or do I stand up and finally make a real decision to change?

When I made that decision, life began to shift – mostly upwards, but also downwards, sideways and in roundabouts too.

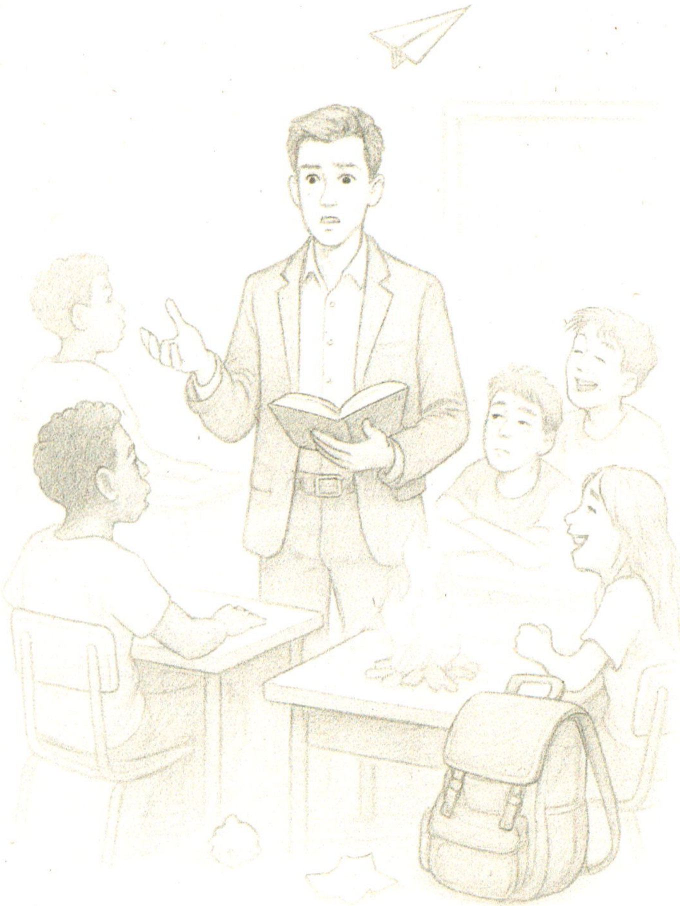

2. Posh Cunt

My third year at university was a complete waste of time in terms of educational value.

But one of the things I did to try to change the picture a little was start volunteering in a school where all the students had been expelled or excluded from their previous schools. They'd done a variety of extreme things – from trying to burn their old school down, to petty or sometimes more serious crime. I figured I could help them... and maybe it would look good on my CV.

After all, I was sure these kids would be able to relate to and learn something from someone who'd grown up in Surrey, in a well-off family, with absolutely no experience of the problems and extreme circumstances that they'd been through. So much so that they had a nickname for me:

Posh Cunt.

I can see how they came up with it...

Not surprisingly, the kids weren't able to learn anything from me, I wasn't able to learn anything from them, and it was no use for anyone.

However, the experience really gave me one useful thing, something to write on my CV. And personally, I felt that's half the point of our education system and many volunteering roles. Not to genuinely help people or achieve anything transformational, but to have experiences to write on a piece of paper, a CV. The key to finding a stable job.

Now of course, there are thousands of volunteering roles and positions that do bring immense fulfilment to the person volunteering, and great benefits to those they are helping, but that's not what I personally experienced here. And clearly, my attitude at the time contributed massively to this conclusion.

I have a negative feeling towards my time through school as well, and I went to what was considered to be one of the top schools in the UK. However, the way I saw it, 90% of my time there was a complete waste of time. Sure, the basics were essential. Learning to read, write and do some maths - things that many in the world only dream of being able to do yet don't have the opportunities available to them. But the rest of it wasn't for me.

I've hardly used any of what I learned at school apart from well, writing, which as you've worked out, I've used to write this book... so maybe it wasn't that bad.

What I really learned from these times, and the way I wasted away my years of university too, was that from fucking things up so much, I could grow. Maybe that made the experience worth it, although I guess there are faster, cheaper and better ways to go about things.

In the UK system, what a university degree and decent school grades really did for me was to show people that

I was capable of following instructions and completing tasks, regardless of whether they offered any real value, and as I was reasonably capable at completing those tasks, and then writing the results from the tasks on a piece of paper, my CV, I put myself in a position to be hired for a job.

And given the unemployment across the world these days, I know I'm very fortunate to be concluding that too. It's what brought me to my first job wearing a suit: working in sales for a company that sold digital mapping data to help companies with marketing or logistical analysis using maps.

The role I'd dreamed of doing as a kid!

In reality, I ended up in that sales position by accident – which seems to be how many people around me I saw end up in sales.

I was in the Lake District giving a presentation on some pointless geography project I can hardly remember. Despite barely having the confidence to look people in the eye in those days, I was excellent at public speaking. It didn't involve any intimate connection with a single person, but a less intense connection with many. And intimacy was something I severely lacked.

More on that later.

When planning my presentation, I wisely concluded that no one in their right mind would care about the project, so I turned it into a bit of comedy while keeping enough of an educational tone to get a pass. It went down brilliantly! On the report it was described as 'Michael McIntrye meets real geographic knowledge'. And at least here I realised that behind all the negatives, I was equally capable of positive things.

After the presentation, one of the professors asked me if I knew what I wanted to do after university. I didn't. He recommended sales, putting me in touch with a company he used to work for that sold digital mapping data. I applied and got an interview.

I realised I was alright at interviews as well as presenting. I turned up to the second interview hungover and dazed after a Tuesday night out at a beer-pong American night at the Virtual Sports Bar in London. Nothing a couple of mints and a quick shower couldn't hide. Maybe the hangover helped take the edge off. A few days later I got a call offering me the job.

My parents were happy! I had a job wearing a suit!

Reflection #2: What I Missed

I think what I missed at this stage in life was finding something that I genuinely enjoyed, that I was good at and that offered value. Or at least trying to find that thing.

I felt like I lost at almost everything, even when things were beginning to get better, because I had no real passion or vision to bring me forward. Something that I now know is common for many people at this period of their life.

But at least presenting allowed me to uncover one thing that I could be good at. It was something I could channel into a job, earn money and learn something from, and it made me feel more useful.

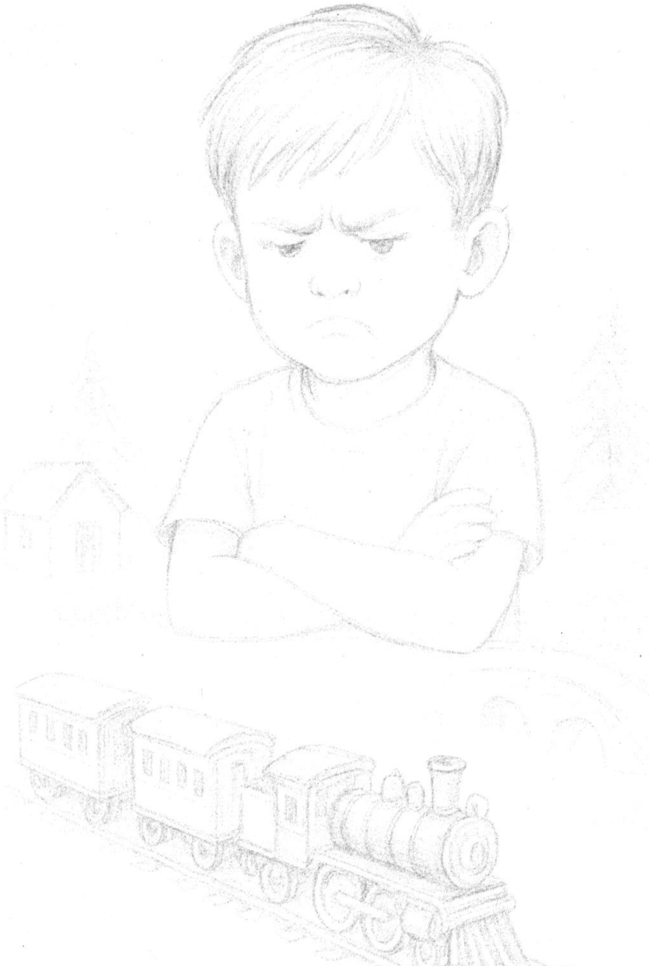

3. Not Becoming Thomas the Tank Engine

Now I'm working in sales, and as graduate jobs go, it was pretty good. It was in a part of London called Brentford, which, in 2011, wasn't exactly on the London tourist trail: the pastry shop chain, Greggs, was probably the highlight of the high street. But I felt important wearing a suit.* The money was alright, I learned some useful life skills, and the people there were great.

I moved into Battersea at 32 Emu Road with my friend Tom. It was a decent two-bed apartment, nothing special, overpriced like most places in London, but decent. I guess things were alright.

As a kid and growing through my teenage years, there were three things I dreamed of doing.

First, I wanted to be a train. *Thomas the Tank Engine* was my favourite programme, Thomas was my hero, and I wanted to become a train. Not just any train either, but Thomas. He had my name, after all! When I understood that I couldn't become Thomas because he wasn't real, I just wanted to become a normal train. I then realised that

* That wore off quickly.

unfortunately, that too wouldn't be possible. So after that, I wanted to be a train driver.

As I grew up this dream slowly faded, though trains are still my favourite form of transport. I've also rekindled my desire to build a model train set – something I used to do with my dad and which he's now doing again.**

In my late teenage years and early twenties, my dream was to just walk – with no money and no possessions other than a tent and some basics – and see where I got to and how I'd survive. I dreamed of walking across Europe and further afield. I never shared this dream with anyone and never even came close to making it a reality. I simply didn't have the confidence.

There's a YouTube series by a guy called Kerr Rawden where he does basically just this. I loved it – even though he stole my 'idea' that I'd never shared anywhere.

My third dream was similar to the second: I wanted to drive long-distance cargo trucks across Europe, Asia... or wherever. I liked the idea of driving, feeling free, ending up in different places around the world and experiencing everything from a completely different perspective. I love looking out the window on planes, trains, buses and cars, and as a truck driver I'd be able to do this in new places all day long. I imagine that after a while it would become monotonous, but I still look at truck drivers with a degree of envy and respect.

** If you're a fan of trains, I highly recommend reading The Trainspotter's Notebook by Francis Bourgeois, the famous YouTube trainspotter.

One reason I never fulfilled my third dream – or came anywhere near doing so – was because it was never part of my set path. My mum worked in finance, my dad works in finance, my brother works in finance, two of my cousins work in finance, and I went to a school where a job in professional services was what the vast majority of people ended up doing. I went so far along this path that I had a second interview at the accounting firm Deloitte during my third year at university. Thankfully, I didn't get any further. My parents were very disappointed; I wasn't. Even so, it worried me that I had no idea what I wanted to do.

On the back of my geography presentation and the events that followed, I'd ended up in a sales role instead. It wasn't finance, but it wasn't too far away from it either. It was a job, in an office, wearing a suit.

I still knew I wanted more – and, ultimately, something different. I was living my commuter lifestyle from Monday to Friday, and at weekends I never did anything other than go out to drink and gamble.

Gambling was certainly an issue at this time in my life. I was wasting far too much money on sports betting and casino gambling. In hindsight, it was all just another way to escape from how I felt inside – but like all other simple escapes, it made everything so much worse too.

So many times, I'd promised myself a bet would be my last; so many times, the promise would be broken a few moments later; and so many times, I'd end up in a worse place than before. Hungover gambling, drunk gambling, sober gambling, Lithuanian basketball gambling, virtual Formula One gambling, 'betting on ex-Fulham defender Zat Knight to score first' gambling. It always ended with the same empty feeling inside me, and more often than not with an emptier bank account.

I now pass betting shops and feel empathy with the people who are in there at eleven o'clock in the morning as I've been there too. Betting shops are often places where people go to escape how they're really feeling inside, at least that was the case for me, until they leave and feel an even bigger low afterwards.

As with all things that can become addictive, most people can gamble socially, in a responsible way, for a bit of fun every now and then. That's great, and I'm all for it. But so many people – including me – don't.

Gambling is arguably the most misunderstood addiction there is. Because there's no ingestion of a substance involved, it's often not thought of as a 'proper' addiction. But in reality, gambling still affects, stimulates and turns on all the same brain pathways that are activated when you drink or take drugs.

A big difference, however, is that you can lie about gambling and it's hard for anyone to find out there's a problem. With drinking or drugs, after a while you can tell something's wrong from someone's appearance, smell or attitude. But with gambling this isn't the case, and it can go on for a long time before anyone really knows – and by then it might be too late. I lied to my parents – and everyone apart from the people I gambled with – about my gambling for years. Most do.

To paraphrase the opinion of former England footballer and current pundit Paul Merson, someone who's publicly talked about his struggles with alcohol, drugs and gambling, he stresses that his gambling disorder was the worst of the three problems. He once spoke about having felt like breaking his own fingers so he wouldn't be able to pick up the phone to place another bet.

A quick Google search shows the rate of suicide for gambling addicts is alarmingly high. If you're someone who falls into this trap, reach out, share and get help.

To be clear here, though my gambling was stupid and over the top, it was never anywhere near to the level of the likes of Merson. Idiotic yes, but never close to the point of harm or no return. Like my drinking, it wasn't something I did every day; but at times, once I began there was no stop.

Reflection #3: Less of a Loser

Gambling aside and coming back to where I was in my wider life, okay, I hadn't managed to become a train, a truck driver or a wandering nomad, but at least I was no longer wasting every one of my days.

This was a sizeable step forward from where I was before.

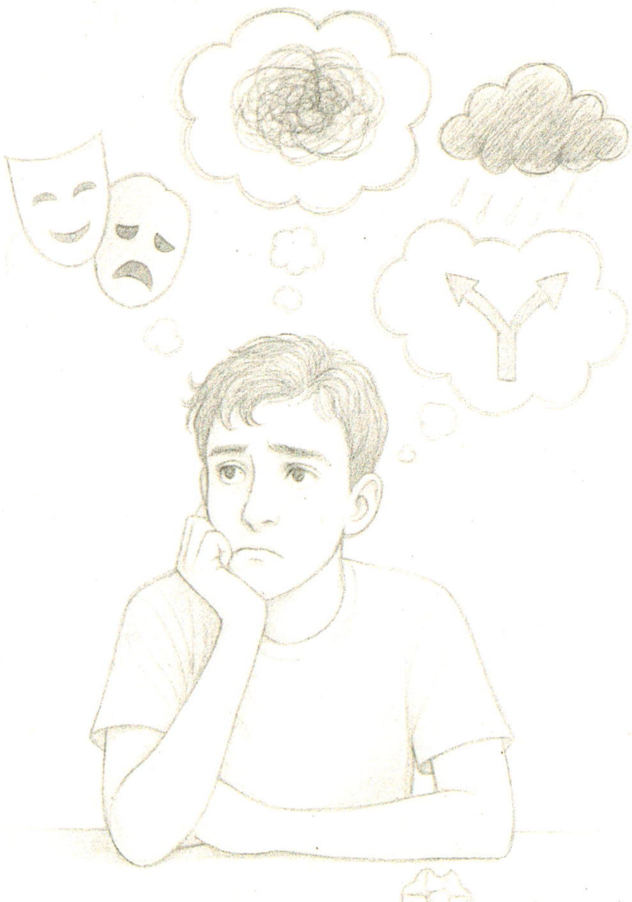

4. I'm Gay?

There's one big area of my early life that I'm yet to touch on:

Sex, and everything that goes with it.

I wasn't really taught about sex by anyone, so like many others, most of what I learned was from Pornhub.

Sure, in school I opened a textbook and the teacher explained some diagrams of a penis and a vagina, and I had a five-minute conversation with my mum somewhere along the way. But really, porn was my greatest sexual teacher.

This is the case for so many teens these days, and usually people younger than that now too.

My sexual journey began at around age thirteen or fourteen with masturbation, quickly moving on to porn. I was comparatively old for this. I'd heard kids talking about masturbation at around age eleven or twelve, but I was too embarrassed to say anything because I didn't know much about it or how to do it. Until one day I discovered it. And then, paired with access to porn, I was addicted.

Combine this sort of sexual education with being confused about my sexuality, as some teenagers often are, and well, it can feel strange when you don't really understand what exactly is going on with your body, spirit and mind.

I now know all this is perfectly normal and fine, but as a teenager, it certainly didn't feel like that.

I didn't know whether I was gay, straight, or between the two. I didn't talk about my confusion, and neither did anyone else I grew up with.

In my mid-teens, I was more gay than straight. I had some sexual encounters with another guy. We did some things, but we stopped a long way short of doing everything. I'll leave it at that.

As a confused teenage kid, I hid this completely. Back then, it wasn't something that would have made me cool or popular at the time.

The encounters with this guy seemed to happen randomly. I guess as a recently testosterone-fuelled kid, I got a feeling, pushed towards it, and things flowed. Our first encounter took a little time to happen, the encounters thereafter continued for a little while here and there, and then they just kind of stopped, and that was that.

Never talked about. Never discussed. It was just how it was.

My mum once asked me if I was gay after a guy stayed in my bed after a night out. On that occasion it was just because there were a few of us and he either slept there or on the floor. I think other people at this time also wondered if I was gay. A few people made some passing comments and suggestions along those lines, but nothing more than that was ever said.

As time went on, I slowly became more straight than gay. I don't know why; I can't explain it, but I know many people reading will also relate to this in some sense.

Past those few encounters, my sexual experiences were very limited. And this continued until I was twenty-three.

At university I once brought a girl back to mine, but I didn't even know how to remove her bra, so I didn't try.

The drinking, the way I was living my life and the way I felt about myself all meant that I could barely look a girl or a guy I didn't know in the eye. On a night out or at a party, I'd be so drunk that no potential was ever available.

I was like many young men at that time. The friends who were closest to me knew my real story (or lack of it) with women, but when I met people in new circles, I'd try and give the bullshit impression that I was 'the man' and knew what I was doing. It probably wasn't very convincing.

All this did bother me, and eventually I got to the point where I had to face up to it.

I was also growing unhappy with my London lifestyle. I'd been working in the sales role for almost two years. Day-to-day life was fine, but I was still going out a lot and not really moving forward in any area. I wasn't doing much new.

I tried doing some yoga and meditation to get in touch with my body, my spiritual side and all that. It was alright, but I never fully got into it. It never stuck.

One day, I realised I needed a change of environment, a change of scene, to do something completely different, feel something different and overcome some of the issues I was facing – issues with alcohol, gambling, women, confidence, insecurity, all of it. In London, it just wasn't happening for me. People often become the sum of their environment and the people they're around in life, and it felt like the environment I was in, wasn't helping me to move forward to where I really wanted to be.

I don't blame any of the people I was around. I'm still close with some of them today, and they're great people. But at that point, I wanted something different.

I'd already been to Brazil, and despite everything that had happened there, I loved the county, the weather, the beaches and the people, and it was reappearing in my mind as a place I could go to – or better put, escape to.

On my way home from work one day, I needed to buy some socks.

It was the day after the 2013 Super Bowl between the San Francisco 49ers and the Baltimore Ravens. I'd stayed up until five o'clock in the morning watching it in an American bar in Old Street. I was hungover – and that's always the best time to make a life-changing decision.

On my sock-buying journey I passed a Flight Centre on Northcote Road in Clapham Junction, and it called me in. This was before the internet had taken over all travel booking. There and then, I bought a one-way ticket to Rio de Janeiro for two months' time.

I walked into work the next day, handed in my notice and began planning my next step. The contract was up on my apartment too, which coincided nicely.

Two months later, I was in Brazil. I knew practically no Portuguese and only one person there, and that's exactly what I was looking for. To start again from zero – or, more accurately, one.

Unfortunately, the one guy I knew there, despite being a great person, was a massive drinker and party guy. This probably wasn't the best thing for me, but even so, he helped me to settle in.

In the airport when I arrived, there was a guy in a Newcastle United football shirt called Jody. I figured I'd see where he was going and maybe we'd share a taxi together. He ended up staying in Brazil, living in the favela of Rochina. He was even in a documentary many years later, *Gringo Favelado*, about foreigners living in Brazilian favelas.

I moved into a place I found on Airbnb. It was a room in a shared apartment where five other people lived, two blocks from Copacabana beach.

This to me was magical: to have the chance to recreate my life.

Reflection 4: It Had to Be Like This

Gay, straight, involuntarily celibate, and being unable to remove a bra...

Some people start young and learn naturally; others don't. Some feel one way; others another way.

And so many people go on similar journeys – though at the time, I felt like I was the only one.

Looking back now, I get it and I know it had to be like this.

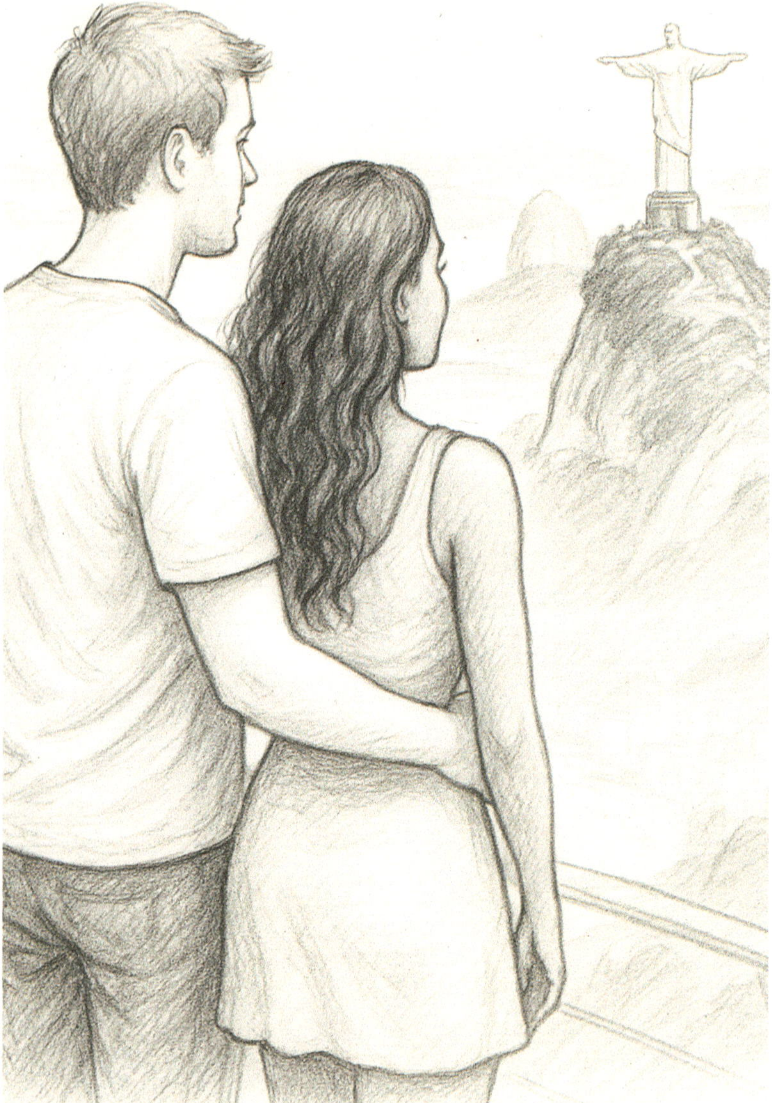

5. Condoms and First Times... Maybe

I had three major aims for my time ahead in Brazil: sort out my drinking and gambling, raise my confidence a little further, and finally get comfortable with women.

That's when I met Maria: a stunning Brazilian woman, originally from Chapeco, who had moved up to Rio from Porto Alegre to try to move forwards with her life too. She was staying in the same apartment.

But before we get to Maria, I want to step back to my first time at the age of twenty-two. Though whether it counts as a first time depends on the exact definition you use.

I was on Tresco, one of the Isles of Scilly, a small group of islands off the coast of the UK. It's a beautiful place with one pub and a little shed (known as the Establishment) where the young people used to go after the pub closed. I was with my brother, some cousins and a few friends, and we ended up in the Establishment after a few drinks at the pub. Drunk, I started dancing (something that would never normally happen) opposite a thirty-three-year-old Slovenian, Serbian or Slovakian woman (I think she was Slovakian... I have no memory of her name, either).

Somehow, we ended up getting together. That sort of thing also never happened to me. And shortly after that, the invite to go back to hers came. A sequence of events that *definitely* never happened to me...

Fuck. Literally.

I'm as lost as you are about how this moment had come about – but as it had, I thought, 'Why not? Better get this monkey off my back now rather than never!'

She was one of the hospitality staff on the island, and she had a little room in the staff quarters where the old village shop used to be. For the whole fifteen-minute walk there, I was thinking, 'Fuck, I have no idea what I'm doing – this girl's thirty-three and she'll be expecting a lot.' And in my mind, one thing I was absolutely certain of was that I wasn't going to deliver a lot. Even the drunkenness couldn't cover that. If anything, it made it worse.

We made it back to hers, and things proceeded awkwardly. I did my best to look like this was normal for me, but I suspect that if I'd been seeing through her eyes, it would have been perfectly obvious that I had absolutely no idea what I was doing.

It got to the moment of putting a condom on. I was quite proud to have got to that point, given my personal expectations, and was maybe even anticipating success. But then the wheels fell off.

I didn't know what to do. I mean, theoretically I did – I'd watched enough Pornhub to know where things were meant to go. But unfortunately, as I'm sure I'm not the only one to discover, watching Pornhub doesn't translate into practical experience.

My erection, which was already struggling because of the fear, self-doubt and worry, was now non-existent – and this led to some of the most awkward moments I would ever experience.

What to do?

There was only one thing I could do in this scenario: I came clean and admitted I had no idea what I was doing and that this was my first time. This led to a short, awkward conversation, followed by me saying, 'I think it's time for me to go.' Thankfully, and as expected, she agreed emphatically – and, I have to say, she was very nice and polite about it all.

But my embarrassment wasn't yet complete. As I began to walk home I realised I needed to pee, so I found a little side track to go down.

At this point, I began to piss, but no liquid was coming out. It was strange – I could feel I was urinating, but there was no stream.

Then I looked down and realised the condom was still on – filling up with urine.

So that, I guess, was what I consider to be my first time. Although by strict definitions, it probably wasn't...

Now back to Maria and Brazil.

I'd been in Brazil for a couple of weeks. Maria and I had been trying to communicate a little, but my Portuguese was almost non-existent and from what I remember, the extent of her English was counting to four. Still, we laughed together, we seemed to get on well, and I thought she was stunning.

I'd planned to stay in Brazil for six months and see how I got on. I taught English to earn a little money to pay the way, and I was planning to get good at Portuguese.

After a couple of weeks, I figured it was time to ask Maria out. I was feeling good in Brazil, she looked good, she seemed nice, and why not? It was easier said than done. Google Translate did the talking where my Portuguese failed.

Maria accepted. We went out the following day to one of the bars overlooking Copacabana beach. This was a magical setting for any occasion. I'd been planning to stop drinking altogether and was mostly succeeding, but I figured that this was a time when I could break the agreement.

It was a fun date – mainly because we spent most of the time trying and failing to communicate in any meaningful way.

I'd never actually been on a real date either, and by now I was twenty-four, so this was a special novelty!

Hand gestures, looks of 'I have no idea what's going on' and Google Translate managed to get us through it, and we laughed a lot. One thing led to another, and soon enough we were making out. A few minutes later and it was time to go back to my place – or hers: we lived in the same apartment, so the negotiation was simple.

She ended up in my room. We got together, things mostly worked, it was far more successful than my first time, and I'd say I delivered a solid four out of ten performance. I was chuffed with that – five or six points better than my first attempt! What more can any woman want than that?!

After a while Maria went back to her room, and we slept separately.

A few days later, I asked her on a second date. We went up the famous Sugar Loaf Mountain. It was beautiful; my second ever date, and to be in this world-famous spot with such a beautiful Brazilian girl was great. We still couldn't talk to each other in any meaningful way, but that was fine; we communicated as best we could.

For our third date, for some reason I decided it would be a good idea to watch *City of God* with her – a violent film about drugs and war in one of Brazil's most notorious favelas.*

It still went well, and Maria ended up in my room again. But I was back to square one.

Nothing worked.

It was an embarrassing disaster. Shortly afterwards, she left for her room.

It seemed that I still had a long way to go to sort out this problem.**

---

* Cidade de Deus.

** If I didn't want to turn to Viagra.

This was another powerful blow to my confidence, and it marked the end of our brief romance. Maria was moving away soon afterwards anyway, and until then we just had some very awkward conversations. It was easier to completely ignore the situation than to address it head on, talk about it or try again.

Looking back, that's a real shame. We could have had some fun together, things might have improved, and romance could have blossomed, but that's not how it happened.

Speaking of the *City of God* favela, I volunteered in a school there through a contact of a Russian girl I knew, Yuliana. I guess I wanted to try and do some good, it was something to do after things with Maria ended and it seemed exciting to go to the place this famous film was based off. Maybe again not all the purest reasons to volunteer and create real change.

It was also pretty odd for foreigners to be going there, but it seemed safe enough and everyone was friendly. For a couple of months, I taught English every Saturday morning. I'm not sure how much anyone learned, but at the very least, it was a nice cultural exchange and something at least a little positive to add to my story as I tried to move away from drinking, gambling and my other issues.

Six months after arriving in Brazil, my visa was due to expire and it was time to move on to a new destination.

I had no idea where that would be, but I knew I didn't want to go back to the UK. I got on Skyscanner and saw a flight to Colombia. I'd heard good things about the country and thought, 'Why not?'

And I moved on as a slightly better man.

Reflection 5: More to Build On

Where to begin?

City of God isn't the best film to watch on a third date.

As for the problems I experienced, again I believe it had to be like this. I understand why now (more on that later...).

There was still much more for me to build on in this area.

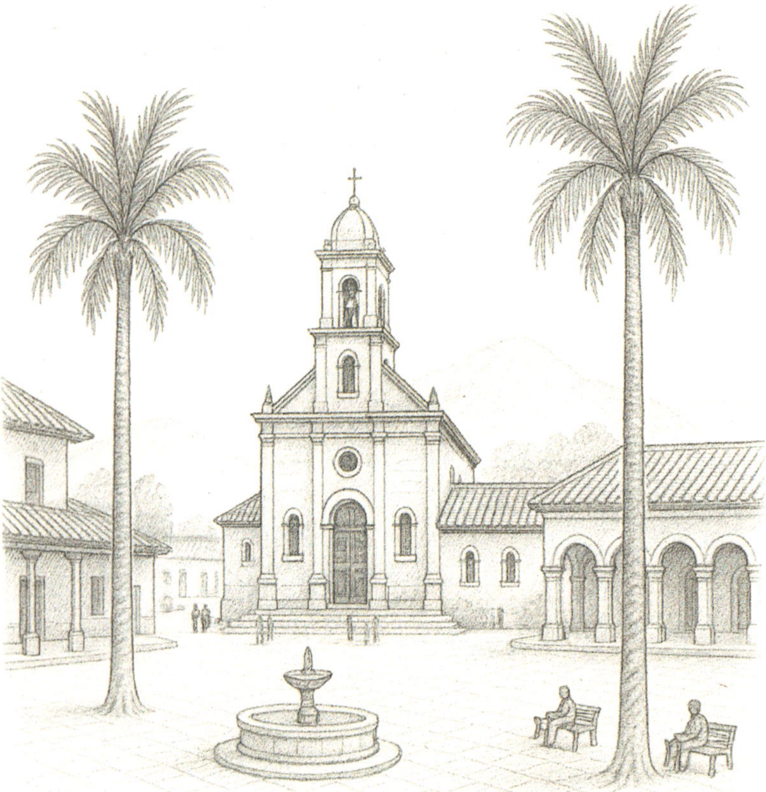

6. An Actual Girlfriend?

I arrived in Bogota airport, Colombia, in October 2013 with absolutely no plan – and no Spanish. I knew I wanted to get away from Bogota, so I simply found my way to the bus terminal, went into an internet café and had a Google about where to go. This first led me to Cali, the world capital of salsa dancing, where I tried briefly to learn, realised I was truly awful, and gave up.

I then got up to Medellin and found my way to a beautiful neighbourhood, Envigado. It was a big stronghold for Pablo Escobar in his day, near to where the prison he built for himself is located, but it's now a quiet, safe and suburban place, and I decided this is where I'd stay. I liked it there.

I went back to the UK for a few weeks around Christmas, did a couple of weeks' work as a labourer with a tree surgeon my family knew, and then made my way back to Colombia.

My aims were to build on my time in Brazil: continue to stay away from drinking and gambling,* work up my confidence some more, and continue to build on forming genuine emotional and physical connections with women.

* Something I'd mostly managed in Brazil.

I immediately met a girl I liked, Laura, on a sort of foreigner-and-Colombian exchange night out. We had a second date, kissed at the end, that was that; afterwards, she ghosted me. Not the best start.

I then met another very nice girl, Eliana, at a house gathering of a friend I'd recently met, who, through pure coincidence in a city area of 3.5 million people, was friends with some of Laura's friends. We talked for a while, I got her number, and a couple of days later I asked her out. More small steps forward.

Eliana and I spent some time together and we had a good connection. She was my first kind of girlfriend. We spent three months together, went out, went on little trips, had dinner – all the usual couple things. Couple things that I'd never done with anyone, 3 dates with Maria aside. It was nice.

I also learned to (mostly) deal with my problems with getting erections. At the start, I tried to knuckle through it again, but that didn't work. It ended in the same embarrassment as before.

I then decided to discuss things honestly with Eliana. She was chilled and open about it. Being open with her took most of the pressure off, and from there it's much easier to perform. After all, I was a fit and reasonably healthy guy. The problem was in my mind, not a physical one. As with almost all things in life, honesty is usually the best solution.

Sometimes there were issues, other times not; in general, things were okay in that area. I was learning. By now, not all my sexual encounters were ending in disaster.

But as my time in Colombia went on, I had decided I'd soon be returning to the UK, and I simply wasn't as into the relationship as Eliana was; the real spark wasn't there for me. All the advice I got was to stay with her until I moved on, and let things dwindle naturally after that – but I couldn't do it that way. Being honest was the only way with someone as kind as Eliana was, and I knew that even if I stayed in Colombia, this relationship wouldn't be long term for me. I was learning to deal with things in the right way.

It was really difficult ending things with Eliana because she was a great person, but it was the right thing to do.

Life was also flowing okay for me. I still felt something was missing, but I hadn't had a drink for a few months – something that would continue for almost five years.

Not drinking is another one of the best decisions, if not *the* best decision, I ever made.** I'd never liked it. It was just a seemingly necessary crutch that I'd held on to in a downward spiral for so many years. Today, I occasionally drink a beer or a glass of wine, but to me, alcohol is the worst socially accepted drug going – and the biggest con.

** A book that helped me to stop drinking was Alan Carr's *Easy Way to Control Alcohol*.

Moving back to the end of my time in Colombia, to find what was missing from my life I booked myself on to a ten-day silent Vipassana meditation retreat. A couple of people I knew in Medellin had done it before, and they had some amazing things to say about it. Essentially, the retreat meant meditating for fourteen hours a day for ten days, with about fifty other people, in a structured environment. It was held in an old monastery in the Colombian mountains, an hour away from the capital, Bogota. There was no talking for the ten days, the men and women were separated, and the only thing we heard was thirty minutes of guidance each day to progress the mediation technique. The technique comes from Theravada, Buddhism's oldest school of thought.

I jumped straight in and was excited to begin.

For a few days I loved it, for a few days I didn't mind it, and by the end I wasn't even doing it – it was just too much. The onus was on me to follow the meditation times and practices, and I just gave up. But my stubbornness and ego didn't let me walk out before the ten days were up. That way, I could finish the ten days and say I'd done it. I hadn't really though, and it would have been better to leave.

The first thing I asked the taxi driver when I got out was, 'What was the score in the Champions League Final?' It was a seemingly random memory that I still have clearly now.***

*** It was the year when Atletico Madrid beat Real Madrid 4–1 in extra time. Sergio Ramos scored Real Madrid's equaliser in the ninety-third minute. I wanted Atletico to win, so I wasn't happy.

This experience aside, Vipassana is a practice I'd love to go back to now I'm more aware of exactly what it involves and I'm in a better place to go through the journey in the way it's designed. I know some people who are big fans, including an ex-professional Australian rugby league player and weightlifter who's done it more than ten times.

With Vipassana over and enlightenment not being found, now was time to return to the UK. But not before one last big farewell on the Southern continent – the 2014 football World Cup in Brazil.

Reflection 6: Honesty Is Best

The oldest school of thought in Buddhism didn't help me find enlightenment, but I did learn one thing in this period: honesty is usually the best policy, with sex, with relationships and really in all areas of life.

Coming clean about my past sexual experiences (or lack of them) helped me overcome a big problem. That felt fantastic – finally, a large weight off my back (or at least, so I thought).

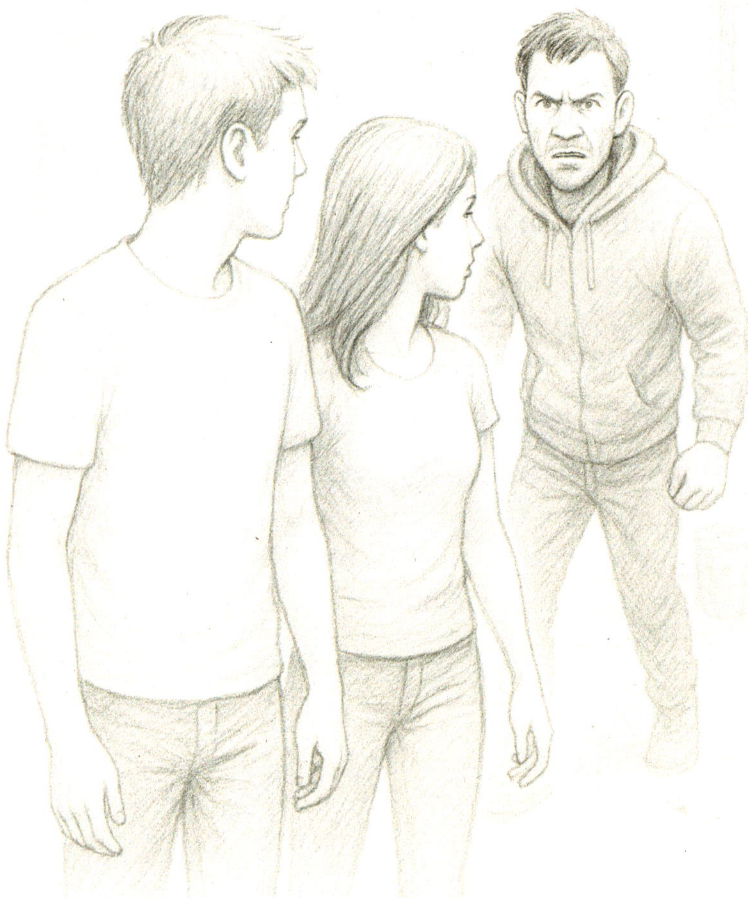

7. Nighttime Motel Robbery

The 2014 World Cup would be the second time I'd been to a football world cup. The first was in Germany in 2006, when I was seventeen. That was also the first time I'd been away with friends and no parents.

Three friends and I had gone to Munich for four days during the semi-finals. We didn't have tickets, but we figured we'd enjoy the atmosphere and watch games from a beer garden, hoping England might be playing. (They weren't – they lost to Portugal on penalties in the quarter-finals.)

In the semis, France beat Portugal in Munich, and Germany lost to Italy in the other game. We spent most of the time drinking and gambling, and we went to a strip club – another first for me.

Eight years on and England were beginning their World Cup journey against Italy in the Brazilian city of Manaus, in the heart of the Amazon rainforest. I flew from Colombia to Manaus without sorting out any accommodation first, and the only places still available were motel rooms. Motels in South America are a little different from those in the US; they're hotels where you take your partner, lover or a prostitute. Sometimes they're nice and sometimes you can feel the seediness, and the one I was staying in was closer to the latter.

The good news was that many other fans had faced the same problem as me, and the motel had become a hotspot for British football fans. It was a weird sight: a load of British football fans staying in a rundown motel, in a rundown part of city, in the middle of the Amazon rainforest – a truly fascinating cultural exchange.

A few English people I knew from Colombia had also travelled to Manaus. It's not too far from Colombia, and England's first game was proceeded by Colombia's; albeit with Colombia playing in a different city. We all watched Colombia play on a big screen in a square close to the stadium, and then went on to the stadium to watch England.

It was an insane atmosphere. England lost 2–1, but it was still a special experience. I was flying onto to Rio de Janeiro in the early morning and the game finished at eight o'clock at night, so I'd taken my things to a locker in the airport earlier that day. I'd planned to leave the stadium after the game and either go out to celebrate first or simply go to the airport to wait.

No one was in the mood for celebrating after the game, but the queue at the bus station for the airport was huge. I therefore decided I'd get a bus in the other direction – into the city centre – and find some food. I could then make my way to the airport later in the evening when things had calmed down.

At the bus station near Manaus city centre, while I was working out where to go, I got talking to a great-looking Brazilian woman, Adriana. I was the only English person there who had taken this strange route from the stadium, and I was probably one of the few Brits in the city who by now spoke half-decent Portuguese. As an Englishman in this part of town, I stood out like a sore thumb.

I can't remember how the conversation began. Maybe Adriana just noticed me and asked where I was from – although given I had an England shirt on, it probably wasn't that. It doesn't really matter.

I still had a few hours before my flight, so I figured I'd ask her for a drink. She accepted. We got on well and after a couple of hours, I invited her to a motel – I was probably never going to come back to Manaus, so why not? I didn't have long before I had to leave, and by now things weren't always a complete disaster in this area. I guess she arrived at the same conclusion: why not? Great!

But the disaster began on the way out.

In many Latin American cities, the centre isn't a safe place to be at night, and the motels aren't usually in the nicest areas either. Walking back to get a taxi, we were approached by a guy who was quite aggressively trying to rob us and who didn't seem completely 'with it' or stable.

Had I been on my own I might have just run, but I was with Adriana. Given that I'd taken almost all my possessions to the airport earlier, and not wanting any trouble, I simply gave him my wallet and the little that was in it. The trouble was, as I realised shortly after, that was all the money I had. I now had nothing for the taxi, and my other card was at the airport.

Even if I'd thought of that, I'd doubt I'd have been successful negotiating with the robber to get him to leave me some money for the taxi anyway...

Adriana didn't have much either, so the only thing I could do was take her out to the airport – about half an hour away in a taxi – so I could get my other card from my bag in the locker, withdraw some money, and pay for her to get a taxi back to her home in the city. Not the best end to the night, but at least it made for a half-decent story to tell.

I told the story to some England fans in the airport, which made me seem a bit like one of the lads – maybe another first!

The next month was both good and bad. Needless to say, it was an amazing experience to be in Brazil during a world cup, but I was still struggling with some things. Sure, I felt much better than before when I was drinking, but I still really had an urge to drink in this environment. It was getting to the stage where I didn't want to go out and drink because I knew what it would lead to, I didn't want to be out without drinking, but I also didn't want to stay in a hostel on my own. Out of these three options, drinking did seem like the easy choice. Fortunately, I made the right decision and stayed sober, although it was a constant battle.

This conundrum continued for a long time. I seemed to associate drinking with having a good time: if I didn't drink, I couldn't have a good time – even though when I think about it now, I never actually had a good time drinking.

I think that deep down, a lot of people feel like this.

Drinking could also mask the lack of confidence I still felt. This is another common theme in many parts of the Western world.

When I got back to the UK, most people almost couldn't believe I'd stopped drinking, given my past. How was I ever going to be fun or have fun again? I asked myself the same thing ... but it was much better this way than how it was before. On that I was clear.

My favourite vice became going to shisha* bars every now and then with my cousin Lucy. This is something I still enjoy today (but rarely do), and I consider it to be far better for you and far more enjoyable than alcohol.

With the end to my journey on the Latin continent, and my confidence (though still severely lacking) significantly higher than it was when I'd arrived, it was time to start 'real life' again. I'd succeeded in my goals of giving up drinking and becoming more familiar with women and sex. But I wanted more, I was always searching for more, and I still felt something major was missing: that fulfilment, inner drive, deeper purpose.

* An Arabian smoking pipe.

Back in the UK after more than a year away, it was time to join the suit-wearing workforce again. I knew this wasn't what I ultimately wanted, but I still had no idea what I really did want.

Either way, what I found didn't last long.

Reflection 7: Life Is Better Sober

Don't go to a Brazilian motel in the unsafe part of a Brazilian city in the middle of the night. Choose a better spot!

That aside, life was so much better for me without alcohol and gambling. It was difficult – I still wasn't fully comfortable inside my body and mind much of the time, often wanting to take the 'easy' option of drinking. But I'm so pleased I continued to be disciplined about my decision.

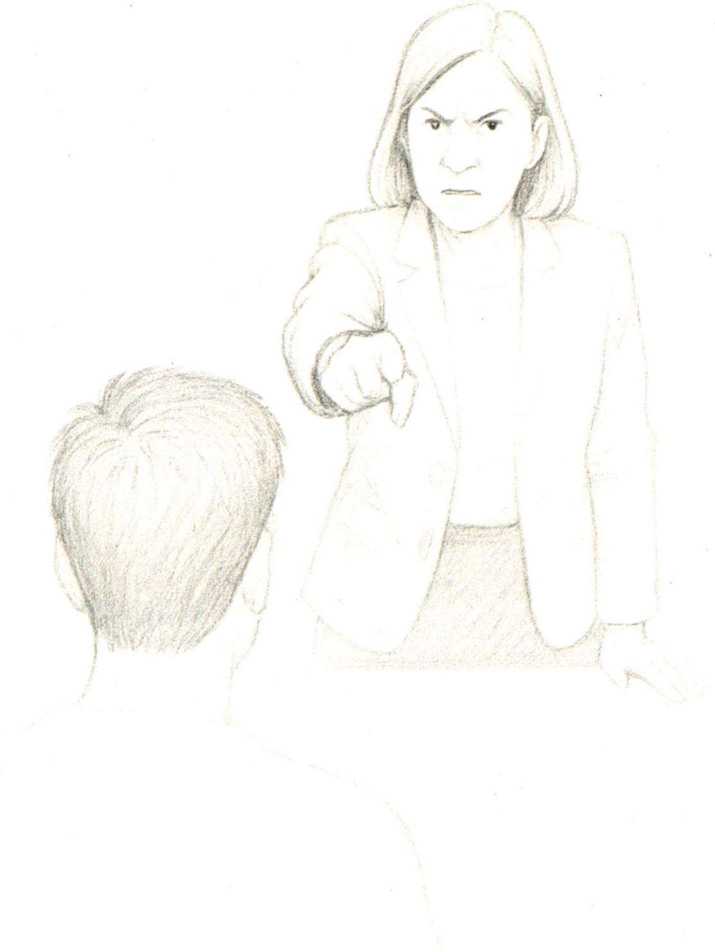

8. You're Fired!

I'd just moved back to the UK.

Looking for my next career step, I figured I'd worked in sales before and wasn't bad at it, so going into corporate charity fundraising could be a good balance between sales and a cause. Corporate charity fundraising means raising money for charities from other companies.

The journey wasn't easy: a lot of job interviews; a lot of rejections. But after a while, I managed to get through the interviews at a military-focused charity supporting veterans who needed help after being injured at war or in training. I accepted the job offer in December 2014, and I was due to start in January 2015.

I was excited to begin. After all, I'd been stuck at home with my parents near Guildford, an hour outside London, receiving rejection after rejection and not doing a whole lot else. They'd been having building work done, and I felt very self-conscious round the builders, imagining that they were wondering what the hell this kid was doing at home all day not working when they were putting in real shifts.

The excitement about my new job wore off quickly. The whole thing turned out to be a nightmare. A *fucking* nightmare. I was twenty-six, living with my parents, commuting for over three hours every day. Outside work, I had no real love or passions. When I'd been living in London before, I'd worked in the week and gone out to drink and gamble at weekends. I no longer wanted to do that, but I didn't do much else. I played a little football here or there, but that was it.

After some incredible experiences in South America, everything felt very depressing in the UK winter on the commuter train. I felt like I was back at square one, just without the substances.

The job was a disaster. I had a terrible relationship with my boss and her boss. Calling rich and uncaring organisations who didn't really care about giving us money unless it would buy them some social points was depressing and demoralising. I didn't have the flame for it – the rejection, the terrible working environment, the commute, feeling like shit, any of it.

By April, I'd already decided to quit and look elsewhere – I just wanted to work out what to do next before I left. But I'd already been called into HR once about my performance, and when it happened again a few weeks later, that was the final goodbye from their side.

It was more than fair, and it was what I deserved. It also felt like a movie. I was told to go to my desk, clear my things, not say anything to anyone and just leave the office. I didn't know it actually happened like that until it happened to me.

I felt sad; it was another punch in the face. I tried to laugh it off with my friends, but to most people, my family included, I lied and said I'd quit. Underneath it all, even though nothing in the role was working out for the charity or for me, I knew the organisation did do some great things. If my attitude and headspace had been better, I could have contributed a little and helped some people who really needed it. Instead, I achieved nothing and cost the organisation money. Another fully deserved low point. It seemed that I was now further back than square one.

I saw one of my former bosses in the street in London a year or so later. I was still too embarrassed to look them in the eye, so I kept my head low, turned in the other direction and walked away before they saw me.

I had to try to get back up. Back in December, I'd had a good interview for a fundraising role at a microloan organisation supporting people in rural poverty, mostly in India. Though I'd fallen at the last hurdle and hadn't got the full-time job, they'd asked me if I'd consider a smaller, part-time role that was open at the time. I'd turned it down for the full-time role at the military organisation.

After the firing, I called this organisation again. They had some small, one-off things that needed doing, and I decided I'd go and help, basically on a volunteer level with a small pay each day. At least this kept me busy for a couple of months. It also made me feel a tiny bit less useless and helped make it easier to tell my parents that

I'd 'quit' my job. I told them I'd immediately found this new role, even though it wasn't really a proper role.

I connected well with the people there. I wanted to at least try to make some amends by doing something mildly good, and when those odd jobs were complete, I left with good regard for and from everyone. Perhaps I'd made some slight recuperation from the events that preceded it.

Moving forwards, I was looking again for the next big step, which led to the smaller step of going back to study. This time, it was something that I really thought I wanted to learn about – sustainable development – at an organisation called Forum for the Future, connected with the University of Middlesex.

Though I told myself I wanted this, deep down I knew I didn't. A master's degree. University. It was much the same as before: another way of delaying becoming a proper functioning adult, studying with other people who wanted to try and do good and create change.

I hadn't yet developed the strong beliefs about university that I expressed previously; I was still working through my issues at this time. I still had no clue about what I really wanted to do, so again I thought, 'Why not? Maybe it could work.'

I did care; I always cared, despite all the mistakes I'd made, and deep down, I always wanted to make a difference. Who doesn't, after all?

It was a one-year master's programme and things went fine. I worked on some good projects, learned some interesting things, met a lot of good people, left with a master's degree, mostly enjoyed the whole thing, and that was that. It was far more interesting and beneficial than my first degree, but that's not saying much – watching a duck float on water for three years would have been more useful than my first degree.*

There were some quite strong views within the institution, which I've since taken a step back from. I also went vegan and kept it up for four years after the course ended. You've probably seen by now that I'm an 'all or nothing' kind of guy, and I bought all in.

This degree was supposed to set me up for my big career move into a role where I was going to be able to change the world. But the closest I got to that was a final-stage interview at the sustainability department of Marks and Spencer's.

So, career-wise, doing the degree was mostly a waste of time and money. Though again, I'm the main one responsible for that conclusion.

After I finished the degree in summer 2016 and before joining the paid workforce again, I went to do ten days of volunteering in the Jungle – a refugee and migrant camp on the French side of the English Channel, near Calais.

* Although there could be real benefit in watching a duck. Eckhart Tolle in *The Power of Now* talks of the lessons he learned from studying presence by observing ducks.

There were a few thousand migrants and refugees there at the time living in pretty squalid conditions while they waited to try to get to the UK.

The refugee situation has always interested me, and I wanted to learn more and see if I could help.

Reflection 8: Great!

I thought I was making some progress with my career. Then I got fired, went back to being a student again, and followed that by deciding to go volunteering.

Great!

I certainly wasn't in the best place...

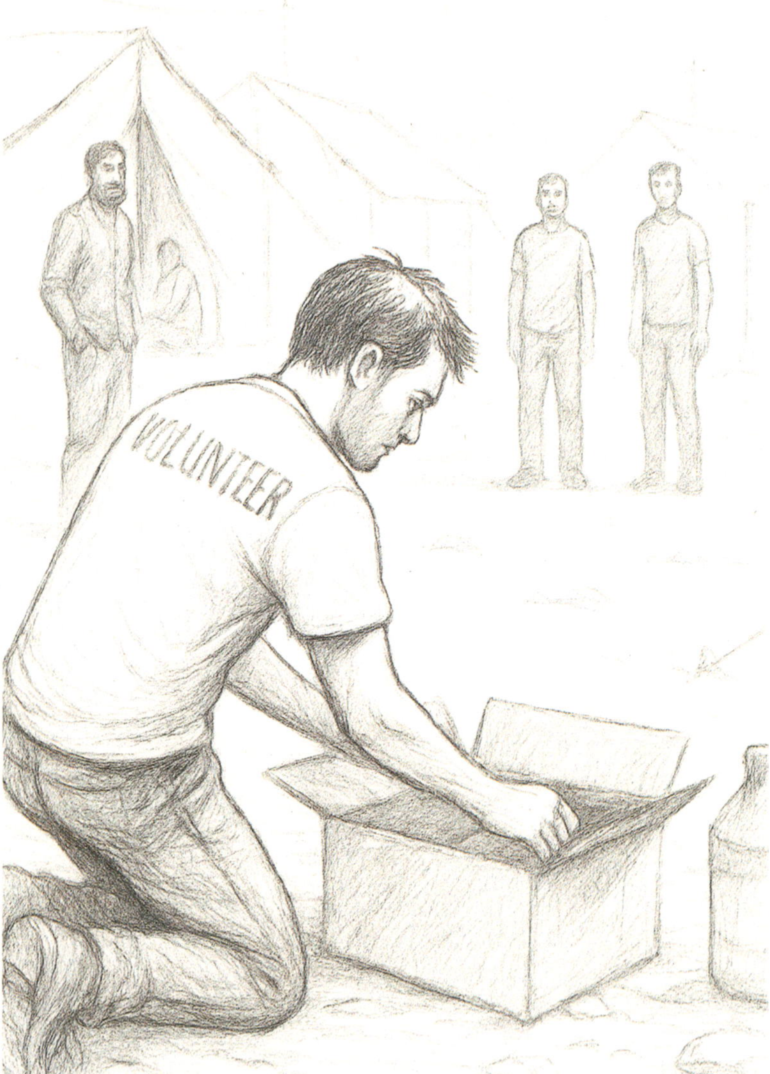
VOLUNTEER

9. Finding Love in a Refugee Camp

I went to Calais with two friends I'd made on the master's course – Kate and Sophie – and a carful of stuff the organisation running the logistics had said would be useful. We were staying in a hostel, and for ten days we'd see how we could help. I was part of a group doing 'mobile distribution' – organising and sorting basic items to go to people in the Jungle who needed them.

The whole organisation, planning and how things worked there was a bit of a mess which I guess is understandable given the situation. Looking back, I'm also not sure whether we were helping or making things worse, both in France and the UK. We were making it easier for people to stay camped in squalid conditions on the border. And to simply allow everyone to stay there or travel into the UK whenever and however they desired would also be madness.

The vast majority of people there were great and always friendly.

However, there were certainly some bad people in the camp. I once intervened to stop a woman being dragged into a man's tent and took her to one of the few places where support was given. I didn't know the exact context of what was going on, but your mind does jump to the worst.

There's no simple solution to the crisis here. It's been going on for a long time, and it's only getting worse. I sit on the fence with no clue what the answer is. If I was living in bad conditions in a poor or war-torn country, I'd be searching for a better life in the United States or Europe. But we can't just open borders for anyone to come in at any moment. Public services in the typical destination countries such as the UK are already overburdened, and there are real and valid concerns about crime and safety with just letting anyone in with no real checks.

Politics aside, volunteering in the Jungle was the first time I got together with a girl I really cared about. Her name was Jane.

We had one day off during our stint of volunteering, and everyone went out the night before to a decent pub in Calais, Family Pub. Calais doesn't have the reputation for being the best of places to visit, but this pub was okay, and I didn't think the city was too bad either. I'm in no rush to go back there for a holiday, but it was nice enough.

Jane and I had been getting on well all week, and I knew there was something there, so I went to the pub with the intention of taking it further. I knew she had those intentions too; she texted me to see if I was coming. Despite being no expert with women, I could read between the lines.

When the pub closed, we ended up at one of the huts on the beach. We kissed. I was very happy about it. The next couple of days we spent happily and mildly romantically together.

I'd agreed to take Jane to the Eurostar on her last day so she could head home. I still had a couple of days left of volunteering. Unfortunately, though, I'd parked my car in an illegal spot near the Jungle and it had been towed away. I then wasted our last hours together (and the whole of the next day) trying to get my car back, running round Calais with no ability to speak French.

Arriving back in the UK, I really wanted to make this romance work. I was completely attached, convinced that I 'loved' Jane and that she was 'the one'. The trouble was, with that mindset it's a recipe for disaster, and at the time I didn't have much else going for me in my life.

I was unemployed (having just finished my master's degree), searching for a job, and still clueless about what I really wanted. I could try and show Jane something different for a while, 'fake it till I make it'; but with time, the walls always fall when they're built on a lie.

Our first date in the UK was in Regent's Park. Jane lived near Oxford and I was living in London again, near Battersea. We met up on a Monday: she was a teacher but it was the summer holidays, and I was unemployed. I brought everything for a romantic picnic, we chilled in Regent's Park and things went well. It was a movie-style date, with me just missing the movie-star confidence and charm. She travelled back home in the evening.

The next time we met up was in Oxford. We walked round the city, visited one of the sites from the *Harry Potter* film (she was a big fan), and then went punting – the activity of pushing a small boat with a stick, Venetian-style, that's famous in Oxford and Cambridge. It was very romantic. We then walked along the banks of the River Cherwell. It was all fantastic – at least, on the surface.

But deep down, at this stage, I felt that Jane was well out my league: 'I'm never going to be enough for her'. She'd been the netball captain at university; she was popular, attractive, had a good job, and more. I felt like I was nothing. The nerves, the fear, the timidity. Cracks were appearing, and everything was beginning to fall through. I could feel it. We saw out the day and agreed to meet again in a couple of weeks – after she got back from a holiday to Lisbon.

All I could think about for those two weeks was Jane, and all in a very unhealthy way. I was wondering what she was doing, what she was thinking, who she was texting. I'd learned that you have to play it cool with a woman, not text much, and leave her wondering too. At least, that's what the people who understood dating would do. Most people learned these lessons when they were fourteen, not twenty-seven. I tried to do the 'done things', but I wasn't very good at it. Sure, I'd dated a few people by now, but no one I'd cared about as much.

I was also having little success finding a job that saved the world, which made the days without Jane feel even longer.

When Jane got back, we arranged to meet up in London. Things were still on, at least. I was convinced she was going to bail, but she didn't. I had tickets to the theatre to see *Jersey Boys*, a phenomenal show. We ate at an Italian restaurant beforehand, chilled by the South Bank on the Thames afterwards, and went back to my house later. This time, I was more relaxed and much better emotionally when I was with her. But sexually, I was terrified of the old problems returning. Not now, not with this girl!

So, I finally went for the obvious solution, something so many people had suggested to me before: Viagra – or, in my case, Cialis, which is a similar drug. I'd always stayed away from it because I didn't want to be dependent on a chemical and because it had a stigma (although less of a stigma than the one of nothing working). Now, it was time to give in. When I look back, I'm shocked I hadn't tried it sooner. After all I had tried and was dependant on worse substances.

I also didn't want to be honest with Jane. I was too scared and too attached. I was too worried about her finding out who I really was (or wasn't). So much for reflecting that honesty is the best way – fuck me, I still had a lot to learn!

I didn't have any experience of Cialis, so I thought it would be best to go for the strongest dose: 20 mg. It turns out that's a lot, and I had the reverse of my usual issue: this time, my erection wouldn't go away afterwards.

At least it was better that way round!

Things went okay. I still didn't have much confidence sexually. I was nervous, timid, scared, not sure what I was doing. I'm sure all this showed through. Jane could feel it; all women can. But in comparison with my past experiences, it wasn't a complete disaster – and that for me was a mark of success!

To paraphrase Neil Strauss, in the best-selling dating book *The Game*. He says that people who lose their virginity early tend to have confidence sexually, while those who lose it later in life are more likely to struggle and have a lot to overcome. I was certainly one of the latter.

The next day, Jane and I went to Notting Hill carnival with a couple of friends of hers and a couple of friends of mine. She got drunk; I didn't. She was confident and happy;* I wasn't. I still had the feeling that I couldn't sustain this; it was destroying me. I tried with the bullshit positivity. I tried many things. But when the problem is so deep-rooted, it requires more than that.

When the day out ended, Jane went to stay with friends of hers, and I went back to mine.

All my fear, worry and anxiety about this falling apart was exploding. I 'loved' her after all, or at least I felt I did. She was 'the one', but this would never last.

A couple of weeks passed. We texted a little, but not much; we spoke a little, but not much. Nowhere near as much as I wanted to. On her birthday I texted her first thing, but she didn't reply until the evening. Often, she didn't reply

* At least, it looked like that on the surface.

at all. I analysed everything. I had all day, after all. I was still unemployed. What else was there to do?

We did agree to meet up again. I'd planned for a night with a couple of friends of mine in central London. That afternoon I was with one of those friends, Kesh, chilling out in a café near Brixton and applying for jobs, when a call came from Jane. I just knew; I could feel it. It was the call I had been expecting for days.

Jane wasn't going to come that night. She didn't want to move forwards any more; it was over. I tried pathetically to convince her otherwise. Needless to say, I failed, and that was that. Another truly low point. One of the worst. The 'love of my life', 'the one', gone forever. Even though we'd only actually been on three dates...

I didn't blame her; she'd made the right decision. I wasn't enough at the time. I knew that; she knew that. I began to cry.

I still went out in London, feeling alone with both friends. I tried to laugh it off, but it was impossible. There was no coming back from this...

Jane didn't give me a reason that she didn't want to see me again until two weeks later. She then messaged me to tell me she was seeing someone else, and that really was that. I was even more devasted, but I understood her well.

If I'd been Jane dating me at that time, I'd have done the same thing. I really did wish her the best. Instagram tells me that nine years on she's now married to that same person, so it was the right choice for her!

The final contact I made with Jane was to send her an Adidas hoodie that she'd left at mine on the night she stayed. I remember handing it to the Post Office in Battersea and knowing that this would be the last piece of her I'd ever have contact with.

There were two channels I used to try to get over Jane. One was positive, and one was less so.

Reflection 9: What Now?

Well, this was a shit time. Fuck me, I was lost!

What to do now?

10. Join a Cult?

I must admit that for a couple of nights, I slipped back into binge-drinking and drugs – but I was determined to never go back there, and managed to keep my head above water in the end. In hindsight, though, it might have been a healthier option than where I did end up: the Landmark Forum.

If you know anyone who's been to Landmark, you probably know that's it's quite common for people who have done the programme to continually invite you to Landmark introduction events, and you probably know Landmark participants often bang on about it a lot trying to get you to sign up. I know this well: I was one of those people for a year or so.

I'm exaggerating a little, but there's truth in that.

The Landmark Forum is a course that according to their website in November 2025, enables you to 'redefine what's possible' and 'bring about positive, permanent shifts in the quality of your life – in just three days'. It starts with a three-and-a-half-day intensive course, The Landmark Forum, their main programme. Then there are countless other programmes past that which will keep you going back for life if that's what you choose.

In one programme, the leader of the course compared the people participating including myself to global change makers like Martin Luther King. If it really worked like that, I feel the world would already be a very different place, as a lot of people have been to Landmark! But as I can attest from my personal experience, I didn't do the course and suddenly become an influential world leader – or a 'leader of transformation', as Landmark would say.

You may be wondering how I ended up here.

I was searching for the solution to my continued insecurities and lack of self-worth, and I saw a post on Facebook by an old friend who I hadn't seen for a while. He'd posted about this magical programme and included an invitation to an introduction a couple of days later, on a Tuesday evening. I figured, 'Why not?' The introduction promised a lot! And because I was searching for a lot, I signed up to the Landmark Forum there and then. It took me a while after actually signing up, but I eventually got round to doing the course.

After the main programme, I did the Advanced Course (the second three-and-a-half-day seminar), the Self Expression and Leadership Programme (a weekly programme that lasted three months), and then the Introduction Leaders Programme (more on this shortly).

I'd actually done the Landmark Forum just after meeting Jane so I can't truthfully say I used it to get over her, but I definitely went in deeper at Landmark after things finished with her.

And whilst I was with her, it didn't help me at all with our three-date 'relationship'. Ironically, her aunt had done it, so she was familiar with the concept of inviting people to introductions. I did invite Jane to one introduction event; thankfully, she turned down my invitation. I banged on about it a little more, but fortunately I wasn't yet so far in that it became central to our conversation.

I must be fair; I feel Landmark does have some good concepts. And can I really call it a cult? I don't know...

I saw people who dip their toes in the water of Landmark, gain some great benefits, walk away after the first course, don't come back, and are all good. If other people ask them about it, they talk about it fairly and explain how it benefited them. They don't push anyone to go to an introduction. If the person asking isn't really interested in it, they leave it at that. Great for everyone involved.

And I also saw people who stay involved with Landmark for many years and seem truly happy, successful and engaged with life and the programmes that Landmark offers.

Unfortunately, I wasn't in either of those groups.

For me, starting with the good, firstly Landmark did teach me to take on a high level of accountability and integrity, encouraging me to take responsibility for my actions and my life. Something I feel is a little missing in this day and age.

Secondly, there's also a big focus on being on time. I love that! Lateness is one of my big pet peeves! Maybe everyone should do Landmark just so they learn to arrive on time!

And thirdly, there was also an emphasis on identifying what my dreams were – or what I wanted to 'transform', as they would say – and on planning and taking actions to achieve my dreams with accountability.

Although with the first and third point, I didn't exactly achieve much immediately after doing this, and some of my actions you're about to read don't exactly sit well with me now. So maybe I can't exactly list these points as positives at all.

I obviously hold the responsibility for that though, not them. And of course you can clearly learn these three things without Landmark too.

There were some great people there, too. Rather than being full of extremists as some may imagine, for the most part, people at Landmark were looking for something more from life, like I was.

In my personal opinion, what is really wrong with Landmark boils down to two main things, and a third rather odd point I feel like adding on top.

The first is the recruitment model. From the very first day, I (and everyone else there) was encouraged to call friends and family to talk about our transformational experiences in the Landmark Forum and invite them to introductions. And 'encouraged' is a polite term for it. 'Forced' would be too far in the other direction; there's no obligation. Perhaps 'very strongly encouraged' would be how I'd describe it.

And when I was feeling weak personally, I wilfully followed along. In a later programme at Landmark I (and all the other people there) were told to write a list of people we want to invite or sign up, discuss how we're going to speak to them, and even role-play that conversation with another 'graduate',* with them pretending to be that friend or family member who we want to sign up.

It seems very weird when I look back on it, but I was doing all this freely. Or in fact, not freely. I was paying to do it!

I invited probably around thirty to forty people from my life to introductions over my time doing Landmark programmes, and about twenty more to directly sign up. My mum and dad even came once. They didn't sign up, although they did try to express some of their concerns about the programme. Needless to say, I didn't listen.

Out of those people, my cousin (who looked up to me) did sign up and attend three courses, and a person I knew in Colombia signed up but pulled out a day later. That was it.

I wasn't a very successful recruiter!

The second big problem is that the programme was almost talked about by Landmark as the ultimate answer to all life's problems. I'm paraphrasing a little but basically the *most powerful* solution there is: no other ways work as well, if at all.

---

* Graduates are what Landmark calls people who have done the 'Landmark Forum', the first programme.

A conversation about how to invite more people to the Landmark Forum was once described by one of the leaders as 'the most important conversation going on in the world right now'. Looking back now, this seems just mental to me that I sat here and listened to this without questioning it. There are so many paths to personal growth, purpose and happiness, and these will always be different for different people. Maybe for some it's Landmark, but for others it can be painting, swimming, yoga, or whatever else.

For me, it definitely wasn't Landmark.

The third problem is the way us 'graduates' talked to each other. There's almost a dictionary of 'inside' words. For example, instead of 'graduates' saying they're complaining to each other, they say they're 'running a racket'. I mean maybe calling this a problem is a bit much, but again, it's a little odd.

How did I not see these issues when they're so clear to me now? It's not as if nobody expressed these concerns to me. Many people did, some in very direct ways.

It was because I was sad, lonely, a little lost and weak. I needed an answer. Drinking didn't work, drugs didn't work, gambling didn't work, and meditation didn't work, so why not try this? I was willing to try anything. And after things with Jane ended, all of the above sensations were multiplied!

The Introduction Leaders Programme is a seven-month course that you pay for. In it, you train to become one of the people who can go to other people's houses (when invited to do so by a graduate) to lead introductions and potentially sign people up to the Landmark Forum.

This involved four weekend seminars, a regular Friday night at the Landmark Centre, and many hours spent at the centre calling people and friends to ask them to sign up to the course or come to introductions. All this took place over seven months.

Of all the choices I've made in life, this is among the ones I'm most uncomfortable about. Not necessarily because I did the courses, but how I got so involved in it trying to invite so many people to introductions and to sign up. Telling them I was 100% sure about it at the time!

While I was on the course, I almost bought into some dodgy investment scheme from another participant, Joseph. When I introduced the investment to my old friend Tom, he warned me in very strong terms that it was complete nonsense – but my reply was, 'I trust this guy with my life.' This was simply because Joseph was doing the Landmark Introduction Leaders Programme and there was a big emphasis on 'honesty and integrity' in the programme. Just because he was doing the course, I trusted him more than I trusted a friend I'd known for years.

Luckily for me, one of the rules of the programme was along the lines of not doing business with other participants. I took the programme seriously, so this stopped me diving into the investment headfirst. I was also starting to come to my senses thanks to people like Tom, even though I never admitted it at the time. From what I can now see online, Joseph was later arrested. So much for honesty and integrity.

In 2017, when I was doing the Introduction Leaders Programme, the criteria for becoming an introduction leader involved personally signing five people up to the Landmark Forum (of this I achieved one – the person who didn't do it), and inviting fifteen people to a Landmark introduction who actually attend (I achieved my fifteen – well done me! – but zero signed up).

I also had to learn a list of questions and answers about Landmark and my Landmark coach tested me to check I knew the answers well enough. One of these questions was along the lines of, 'Is Landmark a cult?' And I had to learn the reply about why it wasn't, which was about three paragraphs long. I mean, what place that definitely isn't a cult needs to teach people to answer a question on why it's not a cult?

There were a few more requirements for achieving introduction leader status, but those three stood out.

In the bottom of my heart, and in my mind and spirit, I think I knew all this wasn't right for me. But I was so caught up in it, and if you tell a graduate you're having doubts, the reply from them was often that I was 'running a racket'. I was so lost that I just went along with it for a year or so until the last session of the Introduction Leaders Programme. That was the last time I stepped foot in a Landmark building.

There was no dramatic ending. At this time, I thought I may even continue with a Landmark program or two at some point in the near future, but I did have a hunch that a little break could be good for me to gather my senses, and thankfully through time, I did.

Reflection 10: Fuck Me, I Was Lost

Ctrl-C, Ctrl-V.

Fuck me, I was lost!

What to try next?

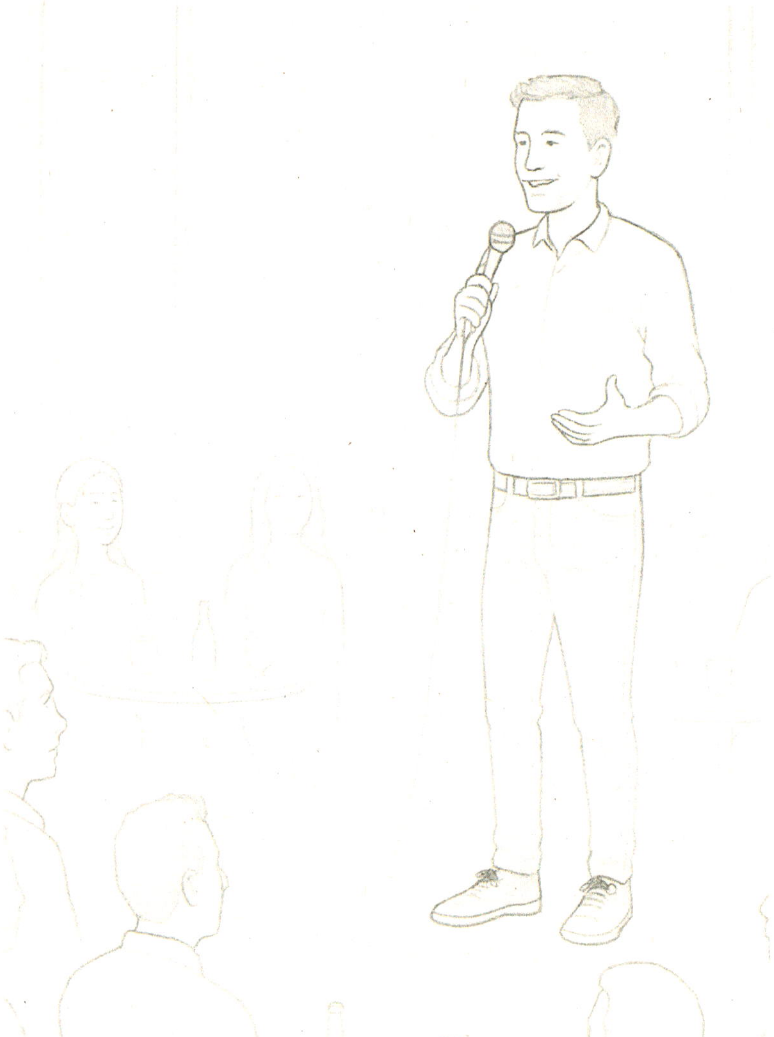

11. Performing at a Gay Pole-Dancing Club

The second way I got over Jane was through comedy.

I decided I'd try a course in stand-up comedy. Again, I'm not sure it was entirely because things finished with her, but it coincided nicely. As I've mentioned before, I didn't mind speaking in front of a crowd.

But public speaking is only half of comedy. The other more important half is the comedy part. I thought I could be good at it, so why not try? I enrolled in a course of 'sustainable stand-up comedy' – stand-up but with a focus on the environment and social issues. I was still pursuing the trying to change the world angle side of things, despite achieving very little with it.

It was a decent eight-week course. There was a workshop every Friday evening and at the end of it, everyone had a five-minute live set to perform. Ironically, another participant, Neils, who was from Germany, had also done the Landmark Forum and included that as a joke in his five-minute set.

The location for the set was in the basement of a gay pole-dancing club in Soho, London. I'd made it!

As you might have guessed, there were no gay pole-dancers when we were there.

I delivered a five-minute set, and it got a pretty good reception. I wasn't going to get invited to the Apollo any time soon, but there were enough laughs to give me hope.

And because I'd had one half-decent five-minute comedy slot in a controlled location where I invited a few friends and my brother, I thought I'd keep going until I made the top.

In total I did around twenty different shows, all in walk-on or free sign-up events at random depressing bars and dark clubs across London. I had some great shows, once almost winning 'comedian of the night' as one of fifteen other people. I also had a few really terrible shows, with barely a laugh. It's a strange experience – standing on stage trying to make people laugh and watching zero people laugh back at you.

I even dreamed of becoming a full-time comedian, given all the success I'd had on Tuesday nights in half-empty bars. I listed my job role on LinkedIn as 'Comedian, Creator, Conservation' – whatever the fuck that's meant to mean.

I went up to the Edinburgh Festival: the biggest comedy festival in the UK and one of the biggest in the world. I had intended to perform at free sign-up shows, but they were already full, so instead I spent the few days going along to events. And I left it there. That was that for my career in comedy. I lost the vision for it quickly.

Doing comedy in front of people helped build my confidence back, filled some time and eased the strain I was feeling. That was certainly a good thing.

But I was still lost. I still hadn't found my mission and I still wanted more, and I wasn't finding that in London.

By then, I was back at work. I spent three or four months with the environmental organisation WWF as a project intern earning the national living wage. Jesus – to get my foot in the door to a job trying to save the world, because I'd had no success at any other organisation, I was now a twenty-eight-year-old intern. I helped to promote a campaign called 'Earth Hour'– essentially a night where for an hour in one evening in March or April, people at home, as well as major monuments, government buildings and corporate offices, turn off all their lights for one hour to supposedly raise awareness about climate change.

It was better than sitting at home failing to find a real job whilst wondering what the hell I was doing.

After Earth Hour finished, I moved on to do some work with Diabetes UK as a temporary project manager. The purpose of the temporary role was to help smooth the transition from one permanent manager to the next. I'd been second choice for the permanent role at the interview, but the first choice needed a couple of months before he could start, so I stepped in to cover it. It was a proper, fully paid role for that period, but I still wasn't getting far with my dreams.

The best part was the commute to the office from Battersea. I was always a keen commuting cyclist, and I used to love taking the cycle path all the way along the River Thames to Aldgate. Even in the rain, I was happy to hop on my bike.

That aside, at best it all felt like I was moving sideways in my life, at worst backwards. But as with many magical moments, it was during this rudderless time that my life was suddenly about to be turned upside down. My contract was coming to an end at Diabetes UK; the Introduction Leaders Programme was coming to an end at Landmark, and I was getting very restless to sort something proper out.

It was then I happened to stumble across a post on LinkedIn.

Reflection 11: Thank God

Thank God for that post. Thank God for Mikey!

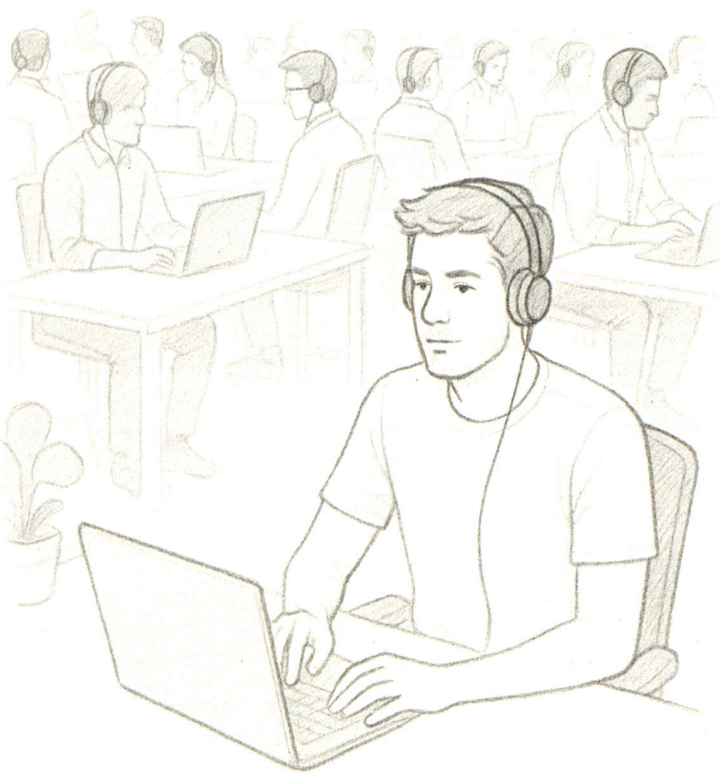

12. Sales Outsourcing – My Dreams Finally Come True!

It was a post from Mikey – who I first met as an eighteen-year-old in South Africa. We'd been doing one of those charity volunteering programmes where you teach football to kids in townships. (My apologies for yet another volunteering story.) We didn't do much teaching, but the kids were happy to have someone there who had a football. For that reason alone, it was one of my more successful volunteering roles, because with a football, we could at least make the kids happy, and that part was nice.

This was the year between school and university: my gap year. I spent six months working as a labourer on a building site to save up money to volunteer and travel. To this day, that was one of the best jobs I ever had – being outside, being active, moving bricks around, working with good people. I really enjoyed it, and it beats sitting at a desk. At lunchtime, we used to gamble on a card game that involved very little skill, putting a 10p* stake on each round.

Alongside my labouring job I worked on the European Golf Tour, Europe's top golf organisation. From Wednesday to Sunday for four events – in Spain, Germany, Ireland

* *Around 0.13 USD

and Scotland – I went to professional golf tournaments and pointed a laser where the golf ball landed, so the TV crews could then show it on a virtual map of the hole. They paid for all my accommodation and travel, a £250 salary and £150 extra for general needs, and I watched golf and lasered golf balls. Again, I was outside, walking round in a fun atmosphere, travelling around Europe being paid, and there was a community vibe to it. That was in 2007, and I watched Rory McIlroy initially burst onto the scene.

In January 2008, I was given the chance to travel to Dubai to do the same job at an event Tiger Woods was playing at, but I had already confirmed I was going to South Africa, where I met Mikey. After South Africa, I travelled with a great friend, Chris. We travelled through South-East Asia, Australia, New Zealand and South America, pretty much ignoring all the culture and just getting drunk in hostels with foreigners every night. Maybe it would have been a bit nicer to experience some culture in these places, but hey, at the time that was of no interest to me. Some of it was great fun, with so much to remember, but much of it was spent drinking my time away, feeling depressed and missing home. I went to get my liver checked once in New Zealand because it was in so much pain, I thought I'd damaged it from alcohol. Thankfully, I hadn't.

Back to South Africa and Mikey. Most evenings, Mikey, I and a few others would go out in the wealthy parts of Port Elizabeth (now Gqeberha): the Boardwalk, Brooks Pavilion, Toby Joe's; all nice bars, well away from the township.

It was a completely different world. We'd spend a lot of money that could have been better spent elsewhere.

The South African and West Indies cricket team once turned up to Toby Joe's after a game in Port Elizabeth. I bought myself and Makhaya Ntini, one of South Africa's greatest cricketers, a Stroh Rum, a type of rum with an 80% alcohol content. He took it fine; I had to go outside, where I proceeded to throw up over the balcony and then get thrown out.

After a couple months in South Africa, the volunteering ended and Mikey and I went our separate ways. Later that year, we ended up at the same university – but for those three years we never really saw each other.

It wasn't until 2015 when we got back in touch. I'd quit drinking, and Mikey had heard about it. He was looking to do the same, and he was amazed that I'd done it, given my past. He was one of the most supportive people when it came to my decision to quit. We met up in London and had dinner at a Japanese place in Soho.

We talked about everything. Mikey was a keen traveller, and he was thinking of going to Colombia for a few months because he was working on a renewable energy project there. Given that I'd been there a year before, I gave him as much advice as I could about moving out there, and we stayed in touch.

The renewable energy project didn't take off, and Mikey began working as a marketing manager at an American sales outsourcing company in Medellin. When I saw his post on LinkedIn, it was a year or so after we met up for that dinner. They were looking for copywriters! And one of the things I do well is write. Hopefully you feel that way given that you're reading this book and you've made it this far...

So, there I was, with a master's degree in sustainable development and a bachelor's degree in geography, with my dreams of working for an organisation that would change the world, reading a post about a job in copywriting for a sales outsourcing company in Medellin, Colombia.

It was perfect!

When people ask me about Colombia, I can never truly put my finger on it, but Colombia has always been good to me. Colombia feels like home. It's where I've sorted out many of my problems in life; it's where I feel happiest; it's beautiful; and it's home to amazing nature, brilliant people, a great climate, and so much more.

It's where I finally sorted my drinking out. It's where I had my first girlfriend and my first successful sexual experiences. It's where I began to raise my confidence. In short, it's the country that's had the biggest positive influence on my life.

For many people, Colombia is associated with images of cocaine and Pablo Escobar. While influence of these demons still remains, a huge part is well in the past.

Colombia has moved on. To me it's one of the most magical places – if not the most magical place – in the world. Of course, with many problems still to overcome too.

I trusted Mikey, and I liked writing. When I spoke to the founders of the company – two people of Jewish descent who had grown up in the States – I got on well with them. The pay, although nowhere near the equivalent in London, was still more than enough to make a decent living in Colombia. When I moved into a half-decent shared two-bedroomed apartment in a nice neighbourhood in 2017, my rent was 600,000 pesos – that's £107. You couldn't get close to renting a shoebox for that in London, and in Colombia it included all the services too.

Given the struggles I was facing in London – trying to find the right role, moving on from Landmark, and still getting over my relationship that lasted for just three dates – it was the perfect opportunity to get back there and start living life again.

I got in touch with Mikey, had a couple of chats and interviews, wrote a test article, and within the space of a few days I was offered a role. I accepted immediately, booked a flight to Colombia for a month later and sorted out my loose ends in the UK. Three years on from when I last left in 2014, there I was again. Back in a little shared apartment only a couple of blocks away from where I used to live in Envigado. I'd found the room through the equivalent of Spare Room in Colombia. My housemate was a girl called Laura; she was from Bogota, and we got on well. She was a great person and easy to live with. After a few months we adopted a cat together, Tiara.

I was happy. I felt at home again!

On the bus from the airport down to Medellin, I got talking to another girl from Bogota who lived in Envigado: Andia. We shared a taxi from the bus stop to Envigado, I got her number, and we ended up dating for a couple of months. The Cialis still took care of my erectile worries, and things were okay. I'd fully given in to the easy option of medication. Although it ended a bit sourly with her, it was a nice start to life back in Colombia.

Work was also good. Although it wasn't exactly my dream role or company, the people were great, the job was rewarding and we did some good things. I was around employee number thirty, and by the time I left we'd grown to well over one hundred people. I began as a copywriter, and took over as marketing manager from Mikey a few months later when he moved up to a more senior role. Over almost three years there I became director of marketing, then vice president of marketing.

I got to travel to San Francisco twice for conferences; that was one of the most bizarre places I've been to. One of those was for the world's biggest sales conference – Dreamforce – and there was almost no accommodation available. Mikey and I managed to find a reasonably priced place in the neighbourhood of Tenderloin. We soon learned why the room was so affordable. It was like a zombie apocalypse outside the window, with needles, heroin, fentanyl, and more. I never felt in danger; the people were so far gone that they hardly noticed we were there. I'm led to believe it's significantly worse now. This is heartbreaking in a city of such wealth. And we were there, almost part of the problem, walking a few blocks away to a multi-million-dollar sales conference.

My employers valued me, I valued them, and we achieved some good things together. My parents were delighted that I'd settled down, found a real job and was making something of myself again. I found I was quite good at some things – sales, marketing, connections, project management. I was never a true expert, but I could always connect dots together, organise stuff, and make things work when I put my mind to it.

Reflection 12: My Happy Place

Come to Colombia and sort your bad habits out! Drinking, drugs and stagnation in life... This can be done anywhere of course, but for me, much of it happened here.

It's probably not what many associate with Colombia after seeing shows like *Narcos* and knowing the country's history. But I know so many people who've turned their lives around in the most positive way, turned their backs on drink and cocaine, and now live clean, healthy lives in Medellin.

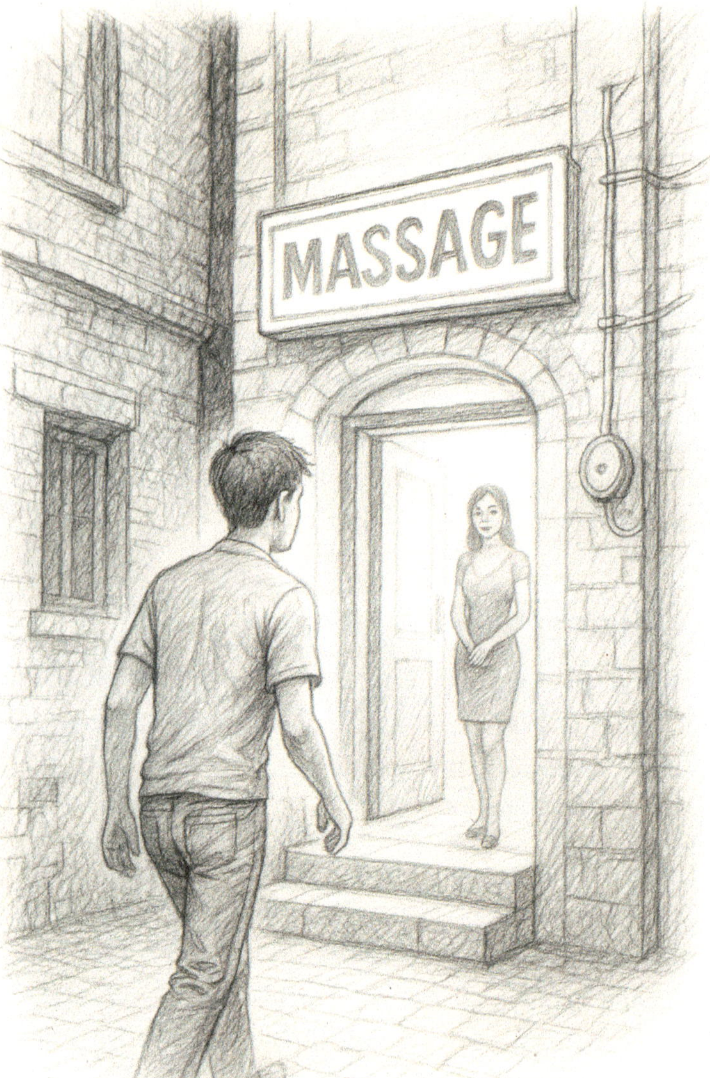
MASSAGE

13. Prostitution

Away from work, things were also okay. I was training (mostly CrossFit), though I still wasn't building any muscle. I'd always been thin, I was still vegan and I wasn't eating right.

It is possible to put on weight, muscle and be healthy as a vegan if you have the right knowledge, plan and discipline. Back then, I didn't have that.

In general, I was still living a reasonably good life. No drinking, no gambling, a decent apartment, a nice job, a cat shared with Laura. I liked Colombia. I guess I was working my way towards the house and the white picket fence.

But I still didn't feel fulfilled. I always felt like something was missing. And there was something I'd slipped into that I certainly wasn't proud of:

Prostitution.

Quite the jump from writing about veganism...

I visited prostitutes on a handful of occasions. The first time I'd done this was right at the end of my time in London, when I was very lost. I continued in Colombia, when I was still feeling a little lost and lonely.

Needless to say, visiting prostitutes helped solve none of those problems. Like all cheap vices that provide an instant thrill and a hit of dopamine, it only made them worse.

As a side note, I never had trouble with erections when I was with prostitutes. Probably because there was no emotional connection and no mental pressure.

With prostitution, I'm not against it if it's done as an empowered and free choice by the woman (or man), and they're treated respectfully by their clients.

Unfortunately, however, it's rarely a free choice. Some people are forced into it because of their utterly dire economic circumstances; others end up there through control, drugs and trafficking. Sometimes it's hard to know exactly what the situation is.

Many people visiting prostitutes treat them with no respect whatsoever – or better put, treat them like shit.

This was not me. I was polite to the women I visited. Does this make it okay?

Maybe; maybe not.

In my view because I had no way of ever truly knowing if the women were working in a free and empowered way (and sometimes I had a hunch they weren't), then no, it wasn't okay.

I knew this and I always felt terrible afterwards. Though it seems I didn't feel terrible enough to stop going.

To add to my hypocrisy, visiting prostitutes is something I never admitted to anyone. However, I did know one or two people who did say that they visited prostitutes. Behind their backs, I talked about what they did as if it wasn't right and as if they were seedy, bad people, when I had done the same thing.

It was utterly shameless and hypocritical.

I now find it difficult to openly admit to visiting prostitutes, wanting to hide this part of my life, but it's part of my story, and I know that for many others, it's part of their story as well. It would be wrong for me to not come clean.

Reflection 13: Still a Lot to Learn

If you're doing anything in life, honesty and owning it are always the best way, even if what you're doing isn't something to be proud of.

Two steps forward, two steps back, one sideways, go in a roundabout, and repeat.

Still a lot to learn!

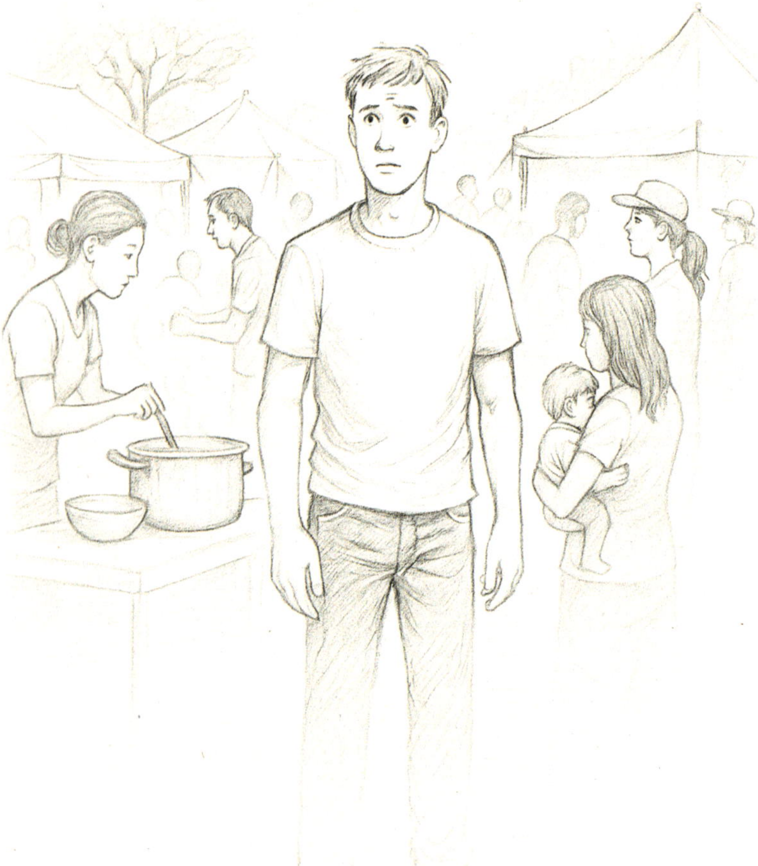

14. Finding Love in a Refugee Camp (Again)

Back to the wider story. I knew I wanted something more than the sales outsourcing role and the white picket fence, and I definitely didn't want to visit prostitutes. I wanted to do something that made a difference and fulfilled me too.

Clearly, I wasn't finding it – and I was taking a few backward turns along the way.

There were also major problems in Venezuela in 2019. Thousands of people were fleeing Nicolás Maduro's regime in search of a better life, and most of them ended up in Colombia. I wanted to understand this more. I'd also seen a Vox YouTube documentary filmed in Cucuta, the main crossing point on the Venezuelan–Colombian border. I decided to travel there and see what was going on for myself.

And as I'd managed to solve the border crisis with my ten days' volunteering in Calais, maybe I could do the same here!

Rather than simply go and see, I also decided to film what was going on with someone who knew how to make connections in the area. Abraham was the fixer and camera guy's name. I wanted to help, and truth be told, I liked the idea of being on camera and portraying myself as a good person.

Abraham found the places to go and film, found people to interview, and got in touch with a couple of people and organisations who were doing great things to support the crisis. We filmed it all as respectfully as possible. Where I could, I also helped the organisations with logistics or other little things.

I was still working in the marketing role at this point, but this is how I chose to use a few days of my time off.

At one of the organisations there, I met Beatriz, a twenty-five-year-old Venezuelan woman who had been living in Cucuta for a few years with her family, having left Venezuela five years earlier – before things got really bad. She was at the organisation supporting the food and logistics. Hundreds of people were passing through each day, and she was passionate about helping them.

She also liked cats. She had three and I shared one – another plus point.

I didn't ask her out the first time I saw her, but I did the last day I was helping there. It would be my last night there, and I had to. We agreed to meet up in the evening to have some food and simply walk round the different areas of the city, relaxing and having a drink.

For a border city supposedly in crisis, it was a nice place in many parts, and I've always enjoyed visiting places where few people go. Going to Paris to see the Eiffel Tower, for example, bores me. I'd rather walk round the streets of some random local area and see what's going on.

The next day, Beatriz and her cousin came for breakfast in the hotel I was staying in – so the date must have gone well. Shortly after, I travelled back to Medellin.

The two cities are an hour apart by plane, or twenty-four hours of driving over mountain ranges, so Beatriz and I were a fair distance apart. But I liked the idea of this and wanted to see where things could go, so we stayed in touch. It wouldn't be too much longer until I was back in Cucuta.

In the meantime, with Abraham, I started editing the footage that we had filmed. The idea was to make a crowdfunding campaign to support two organisations there and try to bring some benefits to the people.

The first was the organisation near the border where I met Beatriz, which fed hundreds of Venezuelans every day as they made their journey into Colombia.

The second was Marta, a lady who owned a small store and restaurant on the side of the road. She helped in any way she could, supporting any person passing who needed help, regardless of where they were from. She offered basic medical care, food, drink and whatever supplies she had. She didn't have much at all, but she did whatever she could to help. She was simply incredible.

Most of the Venezuelans who were leaving the country to go to Colombia, Peru, Chile, Mexico, the USA or elsewhere had nothing but a backpack and a few supplies. There were mothers with babies or young children, pregnant women, whole families, single men searching for a better life and more. To arrive in their desired destination, their only option was to walk – often for months on end. The lengths they were prepared to go to in search of a better life amazed me.

Mixed with that, there were some bad players who were trafficking people for sex work and more. Here I was trying to help, yet before, visiting prostitutes, I was maybe part of the problem.

Within a couple of weeks of launching the crowdfunding campaign, we'd managed to raise around $3,000. Of that money, 80% would go to the larger foundation feeding hundreds of people, and 20% would go to Marta and the work she was doing. For her, $600 would go a long way!

I loved supporting Marta – she was truly amazing. But as I got to know the leader better, I realised that the other organisation was run by an arrogant and dubious person. But still what can't be denied is yes, they were feeding hundreds of people in need. Therefore, I can't be too critical, that was an amazing feat.

I visited Marta every time I was in town, and it was a true honour to see this lady giving every ounce of anything she had to support those who needed it.

Meanwhile, things were going well with Beatriz. It was only another three weeks until I was back in

Cucuta – partly to help organise the logistics for the crowdfunding campaign, but mainly to visit her. I was still working, so I'd travel from Thursday evening to Sunday. I was continuing to use Cialis to ensure none of the old problems returned.

Over the next few months, we met up a few more times in various places – Medellin, Cucuta, and once in Bogota. But as time went on, we were less and less close – speaking less, drifting further apart – and things seemed to be running to an end. She was a great person, but the passion on both sides had worn off. We first met in February 2019, and by January 2020 it was officially over with no tears on either side.

I'm pretty sure Beatriz was already seeing someone else before January, because by August 2020, she had a baby... and in January 2020 she'd been posting pictures with a new guy.

In honesty, our time together had ended well before our official conversation in January, but neither of us had had spoken to the other to say 'that's it'.

Beatriz is still happily living with that same person and their child today, and I hope she's doing amazingly. She was, and I'm sure she still is, a great person.

It seemed when people are with me, they learn what true love isn't, and then find out what it really is shortly after!

Reflection 14: Trying to Help

Refugee camps seem to be my Tinder!

I promise this was never my intention.

That aside, it always feels nice trying to help a little. It made me smile.

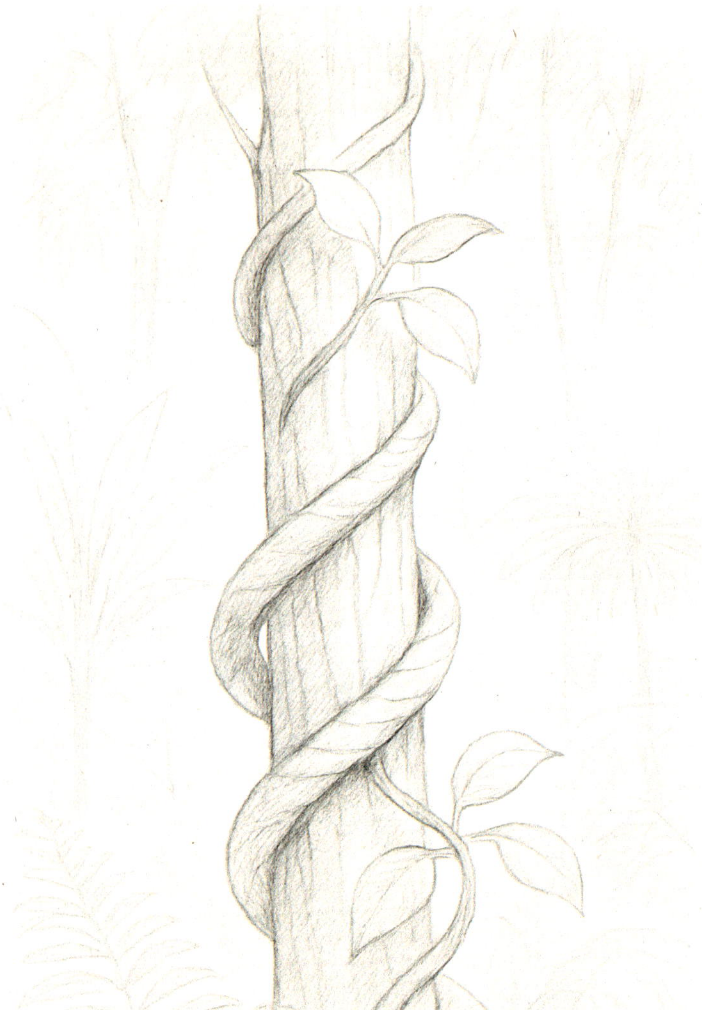

15. The Vine of Death

After the fundraising support project in Cucuta had come to an end, and as things were beginning to tail off with Beatriz, I was well and truly searching for 'what next?' I'd been in Colombia for two and a half years now, living in the same neighbourhood with my flatmate Laura and our cat Tiara. And I was still working at the outsourcing company.

But, as usual, I was getting bored, restless and anxious. On the surface, everything looked better than ever, but I wasn't satisfied with the steady life. I'd arrived where society might expect me to be happy: living well, with a girlfriend and a good job. And don't get me wrong: I know how fortunate I was to be in this position. I'd just come from a refugee crisis zone and saw the situation many people were in.

But still, I wanted to go deeper into who I really was and why I'm really here, not just live a superficial life. I wanted to knock on the head the habits I was slipping into that were holding me back physically and emotionally.

I was hiking in the mountains above Medellin when I made a decision that would radically alter the course of my life again.

It was a beautiful three-hour hike, with some magical views of the city and native forest, and a well-earned meal at the end – all spent with a couple of good people who I worked with. But I felt so tired, uninterested, demotivated – whatever you want to call it. I couldn't understand why: I was doing the things I liked, with people I liked, out in nature, and there was no good reason to be feeling like this.

As I got home in the late afternoon, feeling drained from doing something I supposedly liked and that should have given me energy, a thought crossed my mind.

Ayahuasca!

Ayahuasca is a sacred psychedelic medicine* that has been used in the Amazon rainforest by indigenous tribes as a pillar of their communities, wellbeing and health for many thousands of years – at least since people started telling stories.

Mikey had taken part in three ayahuasca ceremonies and had spoken incredibly highly of its benefits. I'd also known others who had done this and only had positive things to say, and I was hearing about it more and more from podcasters like Joe Rogan. For a reason I can't explain, the afternoon after the hike was when it became more than just a passing thought.

Always one to make a rash decision, within a couple of days I'd booked a place on a retreat just over a week later, beginning on 26 December 2019. I went all in: I didn't just

* Indigenous peoples whose culture includes ayahuasca usually refer to it as medicine.

book one ayahuasca ceremony but five, at a well-reviewed place called Ayahuasca House just outside Medellin. The retreat would last for a week.

I had huge fears as I went into the experience. Firstly, I was convinced it wouldn't work. I'd already tried so many different things to change my life, I thought this would just be another one to add to the list. Secondly, I thought of ayahuasca as a drug – and given my past experiences with drugs, I was nervous about going back there. Thirdly, I knew it was going to be a very intense experience, and I wasn't sure I was prepared to go through with it. But I was up for trying anything, and I did have a glimmer of hope behind the endless doubt.

As I say, I'd already tried a whole lot of other things, so why not this too?

I spent Christmas Eve and a couple of days before that with Laura and her family in Casalinda, a suburb of Bogota. It felt like a place where no foreigner had ever been. It was lovely to spend the days leading up to Christmas with a Colombian family like this. On Christmas Day I flew back to Medellin to get ready for my ayahuasca experience the day after. It was a strange contrast from my past Christmases, which I'd mostly spent in the UK watching *Love Actually*.

When the day of the retreat arrived, I was truly terrified.

I'd done a huge amount of research about ayahuasca, but it turned out that the retreat started with one of the three kambo ceremonies. I knew very little about kambo but was quickly informed that it's an Amazonian medicine that comes from the secretion of a frog.

I arrived at the door to be greeted by Ana, who I'd soon learn was a phenomenal singer. I was then introduced to the rest of the team: Renato and Sabina, the couple running the retreat and their daughter; Darsi, part of the team; and Christian, a great guy and a top musician. There were four other participants too. It was a small and intimate family setting, which put me at a certain level of ease.

Before a Kambo ceremony, you fast and drink a lot of water. The top layer of your skin is burned, and then the secretion of the frog, which has been dried onto a wooden stick, is moistened and applied to the burnt points on your skin.

It's then a short intense experience. Within a couple of minutes, I was beginning to feel truly awful – hot, cold, sweaty and nauseous. I was given a bucket to vomit into, where the water I drank before and during the ceremony came up, mixed with a load of toxins from inside my body. This is a fairly typical Kambo process.

The intense part of the ceremony lasted for around ten to fifteen minutes. After around twenty-five to thirty minutes things were beginning to feel a little less crazy, and I was okay to lie down for an hour or so, rest, and try to regain my energy for what's next.

Why did I, and why do many other people do this, you may be asking? I was asking myself the same question.

I'm not a health professional, and I'm not making any recommendations in these pages. I'm simply sharing my own experience and thoughts, and the experiences of those I've witnessed, spoken to and read about.

To me and many others, including Renato and Sabina, who are both certified doctors in ancestral medicine, kambo is a phenomenal detox and full body cleanse. It's been said to help reactivate the immune and lymphatic system, clean toxins from the body, and help with a variety of diseases and ailments.

I've never been a big fan of the Western medicine machine and pharmaceutical companies, especially after the numerous lies and false claims over the last few years. Sure, if I broke my leg, it's simply incredible what a good surgeon can do for example, but for general health, I'd personally rather go anywhere other than a traditional Western doctor's office or hospital.

In the West, we also often wait until we're sick before we do something, rather than ensuring that the body doesn't get sick in the first place through lifestyle, diet, exercise, and with things like kambo and cleansing the body.

Back to my first kambo experience. It was truly horrendous. 'Fucking awful' would be a more appropriate phrase.

During the ceremony I went through some of the most intense feelings I've ever experienced, to the point where I was questioning why the hell I had signed up for this experience. I was dizzy, hot, cold and nauseous, and the dizziness went on for much of the day afterwards.

I was told this is part of the process sometimes and was given a couple of things to help with it too. There was also always support from the team. I thought, 'I'm here for six days, I'll just go through the experience,' even though I was still questioning everything simultaneously in perfect duality.

We then had an incredible meal of organic dishes prepared by Darsi, followed by a few hours of relaxation before the first ayahuasca ceremony took place at around 7.30 that evening.

I tried to keep myself busy and my mind occupied, as I was more than nervous about what was ahead. We were encouraged to disconnect and stay away from screens, so I decided to read and chat with a couple of the other participants there.

The hours went by quickly and as it began to get dark, we started preparing for the ceremony. I still thought of ayahuasca as a drug, and while we were getting ready to begin, I couldn't help recalling some of my past experiences with drugs.

The time in 2007 in Nimbin, Australia, a hippie community a few hours north of Sydney, where I ate far too many marijuana edibles mixed with God knows what. I went insane for a few hours, was unable to take our scheduled bus back to Byron Bay, and had to lie down next to the pavement, shouting out at random moments like a mad man.

The time in 2009 when I took what was supposedly MDMA** before going into RockCity, a nightclub in Nottingham. I felt magical for a few moments, and then entered into a state of panic and psychosis and had to leave the nightclub. As I was walking home in a slightly paranoid way, I was accompanied for a while by two strangers who, when I shared my experience with them, told me it was normal – something that really helped at the time. I ended up walking round our neighbourhood for a few hours (I wasn't really capable of sitting) until I calmed down.

Back to Ayahuasca. Renato facilitated the ceremony, with the rest of the team on hand. It was a caring, well-thought-through and safe space, but I was still afraid of what might happen. Renato explained the ayahuasca to us in a simple way and answered any questions we had. When it was my turn up at the altar, I asked for a small dose and he happily obliged. He knew how terrified I was.

The ayahuasca itself is a viscous brown brew and DMT is the psychedelic component.

It was my first time trying a traditional psychedelic substance in a ceremonial way, so I wanted to go easy. I experienced some light visions; and like kambo, ayahuasca usually makes you vomit – though to a lesser

** We bought it off the street, so it could have been mixed with anything.

level than kambo typically. Apart from that, the night went by smoothly. The experience gave me more confidence about doing the second ceremony the next day. Because it was like nothing I'd ever experienced before.

In that ceremony I drank a little more ayahuasca. After about an hour, I was 'transported' to this impossible-to-explain abstract womb.

If you've ever asked someone what's it like drinking ayahuasca and the person replied, 'It's impossible to describe', I get that this is a really annoying answer. I used to find it annoying too. Now that I've tried it, I say the same thing. But still, I'll try.

I was in an abstract womb being born again. Ayahuasca in Quechua means 'the vine of death', which refers to a spiritual death and rebirth, and this is what I felt I was going through.

I experienced a weird journey of coming out of the womb into the real world again and then grew – it was like that evolution diagram of a little monkey slowly transforming into an ape, then a human, but I was also growing from a baby into an adult. At one stage, I was walking round the garden in circles, having been reborn into a human figure again.

The colours were like nothing I'd seen before. I could see the energy move between the trees and other parts of nature. I could feel the earth vibrating beneath me. It was crazy, scary and beautiful, all at the same time.

I remember commenting to another participant, 'That was weird,' and he responded, 'Yeah, life's weird...'. At that stage, this made more sense to me than anything else I'd ever heard!

On the third morning it was time for kambo again. As much as I didn't want to do it, I'd signed up to go through the retreat as it's set out – and that's how I was going to do it. All or nothing! At least I knew what to expect this time, and even though it was still bloody hard, it was a little easier.

And then ayahuasca again in the evening. I was feeling better now. More comfortable, more confident, or so I thought: things were about to get really real!

I drank the first cup and waited. It usually takes between forty-five minutes and an hour for ayahuasca to take effect. This time it was about twenty minutes, and it was more intense than any experience I'd ever had. I was feeling every emotion I had ever felt. Good, bad, up, down, positive, negative, hot, cold, heaven, hell, all in one. It really is impossible to describe.

I couldn't handle it any more; it was terrifying beyond words, and I had to ask for help. I was scared of everything I was feeling, and I didn't want to let go of control. Christian and Renato were there in an instant. There are various ways that someone can be helped in these situations; often, what's most helpful is to know someone is there when you need them. Christian and Renato were there whenever I needed them, and that's really what got me through that ceremony. Slowly I came back to some sense of normality. I was more thankful than ever for that: during the intense moments I felt like I'd be 'trapped' there forever.

The fourth ceremony began in the same way as the third. Intense. After ceremony three, the main thing I'd been considering all day was whether to leave the retreat or not. It was just too much. So intense, so difficult.

There were some beautiful moments too. The music and the people there were brilliant. I'd seen and learned some things inside and outside me that were hard to put into words. But for the most part it was difficult – really difficult! I came so close on so many occasions to throwing in the towel, calling a cab and leaving. It was just an hour back to my apartment after all, and then I could relax.

But something inside me simply wouldn't let me go.

Sabina was also on hand to talk to. She's an experienced therapist, trained in the 'human biography' as it is practised by an incredible Argentinian lady, Laura Gutman. This helped me to put a finger on why I was experiencing the things I was feeling, and why I had felt and done so much of what I had so far in my life. It helped me to see the root of the problem and begin to understand it.

Laura Gutman has written many books on this therapy method, and there's plenty of information about it online that explains a little how it works, I couldn't do it justice. But to give a bit more context I'll just take the main website text. 'For over 40 years, Laura Gutman has developed an innovative therapeutic methodology so that each individual can address their own emotional reality, taking into account the perspective of the child they once were.'

I appreciate that doesn't exactly help you understand the methodology much, but when I discussed it with Sabina, it made so much sense to me. Sabina brought out its essence and helped me to understand how I was feeling when taking the ayahuasca too.

After our second talk, it was time for the fourth ceremony. This is when everything exploded in one go. But at first, like at the third ceremony, I was terrified and struggling to feel and enjoy the process.

The thing with these experiences is that the more you fight them, the worse they get. The more you let go and release, the easier things become. That's easier said than done. It took me a long time to release and let go, again with lots of help from those facilitating. But when I did, the magic happened.

I was shouting, 'No, No, No, No!' Renato was near. At one point, he simply said, 'Yes!' It was a simple action, but hearing that 'yes' shifted something in my mind to change that constant 'no' into an affirmative. And at that moment, everything came out.

I began to vomit, but not from tension or fear: by purging, I felt like I was releasing everything in life that was holding me back.

This may be too much for some to believe, but I also vomited a small tumour that was in my throat.

How long had that been there? Was it benign? Was it growing? Or was it just a psychedelic hallucination? I'm open to all these explanations, but inside me I knew I'd released something traumatic that had been trapped inside me for so much time.

I felt as if I finally had my freedom again, my voice again. The voice I'd wanted for so long, so I could say how I truly felt and what I wanted when I believed I couldn't. The voice that would tell me to follow my dreams, to let go of all the times inside of me when I'd felt trapped – when I'd wanted to speak up but had been held back through fear, when I'd done things through pressure that I'd never wanted to do, when I'd acted in ways that had gone against every good instinct I had.

The 'tumour' holding that voice back had gone.

I felt I could finally forgive other people – but more importantly than that, I felt I could finally forgive myself. I felt I could finally leave the past behind for good, that I had a clear present, and that I could move forwards into a future that I was really excited about.

I understood why ayahuasca was called the vine of death. I'd been reborn and had the energy, the confidence and the belief to stand up straight and do what I wanted. At least, in that very moment.

The constant 'no' had turned into a 'yes'. The constant fear had turned into hope. The constant worry had turned into peace.

Why?

I can't explain, but there's a science, magic and mystery to this sacred brew that goes back thousands of years.

Many won't believe it, many won't try it, many will think it's a drug,*** and many will knock you down if you try to say otherwise. That's fine. We all have our own paths, but I knew in that moment that this was going to be one of my paths.

After that moment in the ceremony, the only words I could say to myself, to the others there and to the universe were, 'I love you'. The ceremonies were also accompanied by the most beautiful, most loving, forgiving music I'd ever heard, played by Christian and Ana, and it was a feeling of total bliss to lie by the ceremonial fire and listen to this magic.

I'd vowed to never do kambo again after the second time; it was simply too much. But in the indigenous tradition, the full process is three ceremonies in a moon cycle (twenty-eight days), and that was the design of the retreat.

I woke up the next morning with that feeling of complete freedom still alive. Sure, the fear was still there, but that fear was now my friend, not my boss. I did the kambo ceremony with ease and tranquillity, accepting what was

*** Like I did.

happening, and though it was still tough, it was beautiful. I experienced the cleanse as it was designed: physically, spiritually and emotionally.

Just as importantly, I'd done the programme as it was designed. There is power in keeping your word.

Before the retreat ended, there was still one last ayahuasca ceremony that evening. This was how I'd be celebrating New Year's Eve! I was more relaxed than ever. I still had incredible respect for the ayahuasca, and I still had some nerves, but my mind, body and spirit were all friends with those sensations and I was at complete ease when I received the cup of ayahuasca. I lay down on my mattress outside afterwards and went on a journey of peace and tranquillity. I experienced sensations from the past, visions from my childhood and teenage years, abstract sacred geometry, and so much more. I felt and accepted it all.

Towards the end, Renato came over to me and asked how I was. I felt like I understood the universe in a way I never had before. It was a feeling I'll never forget.

I responded with one of the most hippie, spiritual and stereotypical things I'd ever say: 'I get it. We are the universe and the universe is us. There is no wrong, there is no right. There's just energy and love!'

Although as the years go by I often forget that, lose track of it, and get caught up in life's shit, that's still a moment I'll never forget.

When I came back down into the logical world too, it's certainly hard to truly believe that there is no good and no bad when many terrible things do happen in the world – but in that moment, none of that was my reality. I was in a world that I felt blessed to be in and that I'd have paid every penny in my bank account for everyone else to experience too.

There really are no words to do it justice.

As I woke up on New Year's Day to head back to my apartment in Envigado, I felt I'd finally found what I'd been searching for.

Sure, it's not a silver bullet. I knew I had to change things, continue to move forwards, fuck up, feel anxiety, improve, smile, the same as always. But I felt that I was doing this from a whole new perspective, with a new present and future in front of me. After all, the magic is only partly in the ayahuasca. Like anything in life, that magic only happens if you're willing to go through the experience, believe it, let it happen, and then make changes afterwards.

Darsi is someone who stayed in my mind from that point onwards. She was a beautiful, incredible person who helped with everything and prepared some of the healthiest and nicest food I'd ever eaten. I considered asking for her number at the end and trying to meet up with her afterwards, but I decided against it. It just didn't feel quite right.

Renato had told me that when I went back to the 'real world' my energy would feel different to me and everyone around me. As I got out of the taxi in Envigado to head to my apartment, it was ten o'clock on New Year's morning and people were returning from their parties and nights out. As a stunning Colombian woman passed me, she looked me straight in the eye and said 'Good morning'. That kind of thing rarely happened to me.

Maybe something truly was different.

Reflection 15: The Most Powerful Medicine

In my opinion, ayahuasca is the most powerful medicine on this planet.

Of course, as with all things, it depends on the use and the setting. If ayahuasca is used in an irresponsible way or recreational setting, it can be considered as a drug.

But if it's used with its true intentions, as inspired by the indigenous communities of the Amazon for thousands of years, it can be life-changing.

It certainly was for me, and it also gave me the possibility of faith.

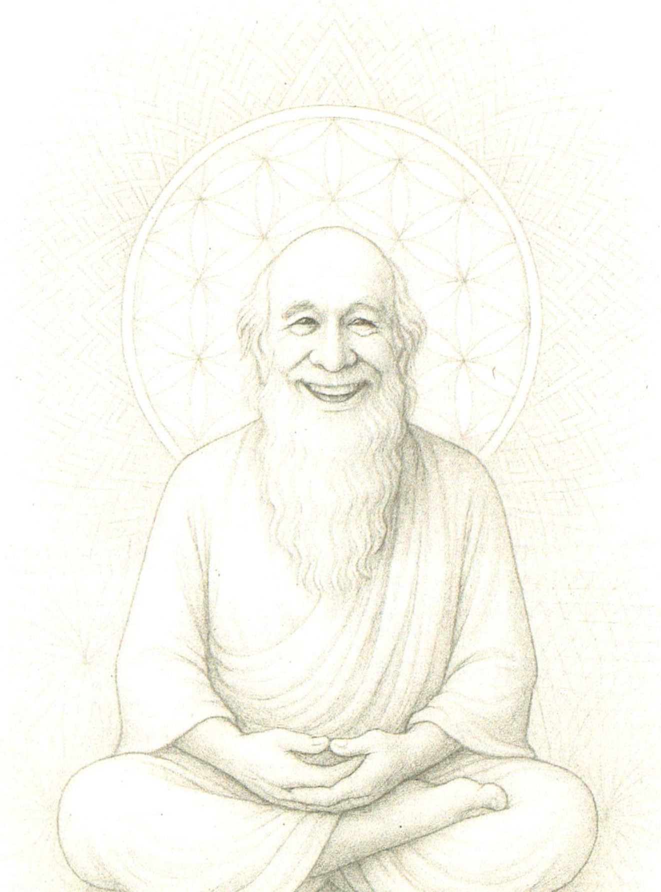

16. God

When I returned from my retreat, I got back to my apartment to find it was dusty and a mess. There were half-dead plants everywhere. Old things needed throwing out, and fresh things needed bringing in. It seemed like the most obvious place to go to start making some real changes. I'd cleaned out and renovated my whole body, so why not do the same to my home?

It was also time to change my diet. I'd been vegan for the past four or five years, and I'd been eating pretty terribly. During the ayahuasca retreat I ate eggs for the first time in ages, and the protein and fat they gave my body made me feel great. When I thought about the fake meats I'd been eating, there really was no comparison.

Nowadays, wherever possible, I eat a varied diet involving all the staples, fruit, vegetables, free-range eggs, a little chicken and fish, and the occasional red meat here and there. I'm much happier and healthier eating this way, choosing organic and local wherever I can. When I do eat animal products, I try to make sure they're free range, that the animals were treated well and that the products are of good quality. I'm fortunate to have these choices available to me. Many don't and never will.

Diet aside, after the retreat I began meditating more, tried to stay further away from phones and screens, deleted my Facebook account, started learning Muay Thai, and took a more relaxed attitude to issues at work. Things improved.

I also started to learn the *quena*: a traditional wooden flute played in the Andes. If someone had told me before the retreat that I'd start to learn a musical instrument at the age of thirty, I'd have thought it was a joke. But this instrument sounded magical during the retreat, I decided to pick it up. I later took a step back from the quena and am now regularly playing the guitar and singing.

The ayahuasca experience wasn't just some instant revelation that wore off shortly afterwards. Life was still tough sometimes, and I still had moments of feeling lost or being a dickhead – just ask my friends and family. But the proportion of time I spent in that state had shifted.

However, the biggest change to my life came through finding God after spending thirty years as a stone-cold atheist. I've seen this happen to a lot of people after trying psychedelics. It's another part of the magic and mystery.

When I say I found 'God', I don't mean religion or the idea of a particular god. I mean a true connection to something bigger than me, you, or anyone. We don't even have to call it God. You could replace that word with 'energy' or 'the universe', whatever you prefer, but I find that the easiest way to describe it is simply 'God'. In many parts of our society, this has now become almost a dirty word.

Before my retreat, I was as atheist as they come; I had been all my life. God was the most illogical word that existed. How could this all-powerful man in the sky exist and control things? I used to laugh and joke about it with friends. Complete nonsense! And that sense of the word is still complete nonsense too. That's not what I'm talking about.

Ultimately, the way I see it, I'm God, you're God, we're all God, and we're all connected. Everything is God, and we're part of God. Us, nature, life, death; it's all one, and we're all one. It's the miracle of life and existence.

And ultimately, that one to me is a great power, a divine energy and a spiritual force that moves us all. That to me is God. I now believe in miracles, in the divine, and in powers that science can't explain.

A friend and phenomenal musician, Gokula, helped me to put my beliefs into these words. Many others find this equally hard. It's often the case for those who believe, whereas the scientific counterargument for atheism is so much easier to formulate and express.

I used to hide behind the 'science' and had no faith. How could I have come to this?

The answer is faith. True faith. Faith that we're here for a greater reason and faith that there's something bigger than us all.

The belief that there's nothing makes equally little sense to me. How did we get here, after all? Sure, the Big Bang, but who created that? The idea of God makes as little sense to me as well, so I get it, but that's where faith comes in.

These beliefs I now express could be explained by some without using the word *God*, but to me, that word gives extra power and meaning to phrases like 'purpose in life' that I could also use.

This faith is one of the greatest gifts I've ever discovered. I often forget it. I often lose sight of it. But when I really need it, it's there – and that's magical.

For me, perhaps another miracle. And for those who are where I used to be, it might be just a mad psychedelic vision.

Reflection 16: Faith

I think I've just summed it up in the last five paragraphs and to add a little extra emphasis:

This faith is one of the greatest gifts I've ever discovered!

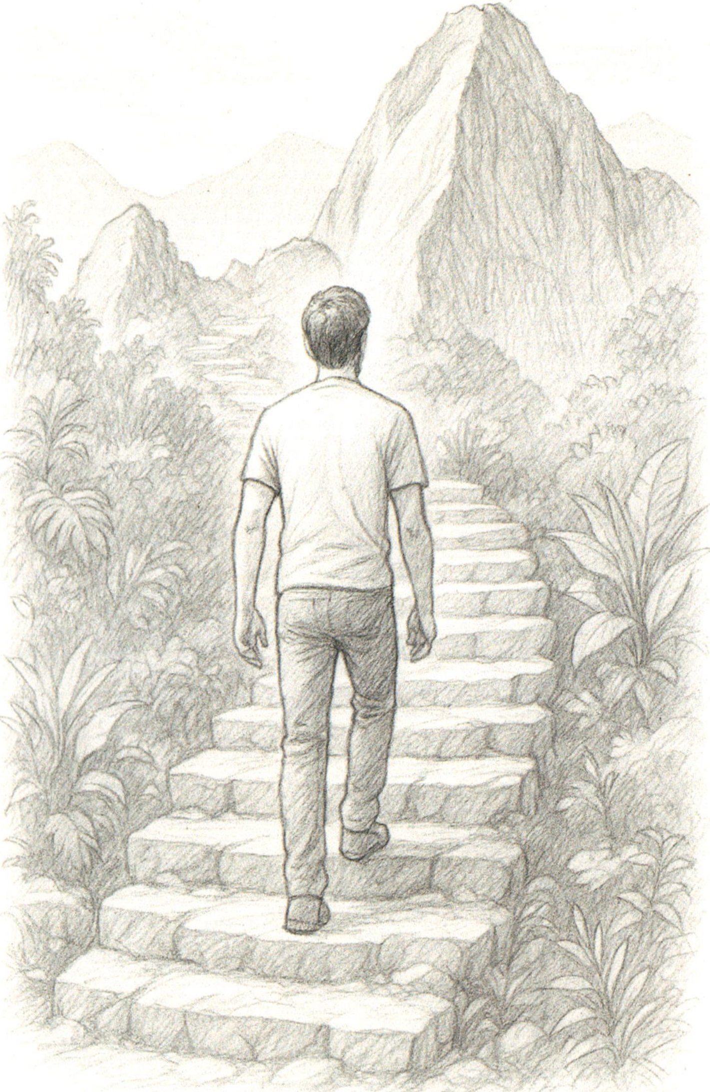

17. The Next Step

Moving forwards from the retreat and my newfound faith, and now more back to the material world, I was clear that my time at the outsourcing company was coming to an end. I stayed on for another six months or so altogether, but three months after the retreat I cut my working hours and booked a three-week trip round Bolivia. I set off in mid-March 2020, full of excitement: Andean culture fascinated me.

Unfortunately, after three days in La Paz, mostly under curfew, I had to return to Colombia because they were going to close the borders because of Covid-19.

If there's one way to make an already ill world worse, it's to lock people in their homes so they can't exercise or get vitamin D from the sun, crucial for overcoming a cold or flu. To cut off people's social lives and community, which blue zones* show is the factor that extends people's life expectancy more than anything else. Make people wear face masks that made it uncomfortable to breathe. Scare the shit out of everyone through every source of news – one of the worst things you can do for the immune system.

---

* Places in which people live far beyond the expected life expectancy.

Call me a conspiracy theorist if you must, but I believe that the reaction to this event was the main problem.

Rant aside, when I returned to Colombia from Bolivia, I was locked in my apartment, like much of the world, for a little while. I was lucky to have returned to Colombia before they shut the border. If I hadn't had an official visa, I'd have had to stay in Bolivia.

In Colombia, I volunteered a couple times bringing food to communities in need who had been cut off from easy access to it. This also helped me stay healthy and sane as it gave me a free pass to get out a little.

Through this period and after things had calmed down a bit, I also experimented with other alternate states of consciousness. One, rather interestingly, can be achieved through the breath alone: holotropic breathwork. This technique was made famous by Stanislav Grof, someone who spent a lot of time examining the effects of LSD and then, after the United States government clamped down on LSD use, the breath.

Holotropic breathing is an incredibly intense form of breathing. It involves breathing in very deeply and quickly, then exhaling fully and profoundly, with no break between the inhale and exhale. Essentially, it decreases the levels of carbon dioxide in your body, which results in some crazy sensations. I probably explained that wrong, but you get the rough idea...

The first time I tried this with a friend, Joseph, who's a breathwork facilitator, I had the sense that I was a dinosaur[**] running through the jungle. I knew I was still on a yoga mat breathing, but when I let myself go, it was also a very real vision.

I really like this style of therapy: using just your breath to create altered states of consciousness. I've known many people who have had profound breakthroughs, visions and transformations in their life after using this method as a central technique. Nobody can make the breath illegal, either!

I did a few hours of breathwork with Joseph to begin with, and it took me deeper into the spiritual/physical connection and built on the lessons that ayahuasca had taught me.

Through Joseph, I also managed to connect with many more like-minded people who were into naturally optimising their physical and mental health, as well as using psychedelics responsibly. He also introduced me to a men's group that got together every Wednesday evening to chat about stuff, open up about challenges and share successes. It was essentially a few good people regularly getting together, and I'm still in touch with some of them today.

I found out about ice baths, sauna therapy, mushrooms, online business, trading, alternative communities, and more. As always, I was diving into all this quickly... and maybe from the outside it all sounds a bit cult-like again. I

** A triceratops, like Sarah from *The Land Before Time*.

get it. After my Landmark experience, my reputation had taken a hit.

Those at the men's group were interested in different ways of living, in a more natural way. There was no pressure to do anything, and I was excited by this new world that felt much more 'me'. It was much more what I was looking for.

This closer connection to myself allowed me to share more about myself with others. Before, other people's opinions had crippled me. Now I'm not that bothered if people don't like what I say or write. You don't have to read it, and you don't have to believe it.

I experimented with magic mushrooms a little too, and I still love doing that to this day. I tried LSD once, though not in the best environment and it didn't lead to a good experience. It's something I'd love to try again.

I was happy most of the time, and I was still a selfish dickhead some of the time.

I think most people around me could see and feel the change in me too, even if it was harder for my friends and family back in the UK to relate to what I was up to at times. It took me longer to fully open up to my parents about my experiences, because I wasn't sure they'd get it. But, as you'll see later, they 100% did.

Everything I was doing was done in a controlled way,[***] with experienced people who knew what they were doing.

*** The LSD experience aside.

They were people I trusted, as I believe these experiences should always be done. None of these things should be tried in uncontrolled environments in my opinion, and they're not for everyone. They'll only ever work if people are open too. If not, it's a waste of time.

For me, the proof was in the pudding (as the English expression goes), and my life was working better than ever.

Shortly after I'd finished the job at the outsourcing company, Mikey had already started his own company in London. He knew I was ready for something new, and he offered me a flexible role, for more money, in a marketing and sales messaging position in which I would be a good fit. It still wasn't my dream job, but it was a big step towards more money and more freedom, and it would allow me to continue working with someone I really connected with, so I took it. It could all be done remotely from Colombia too.

My health was also better than ever, as was my general wellbeing. Everything was working smoothly, thanks to the 'drugs'!

But there was still always one thing missing that I really wanted: a girlfriend, or better put, a true-life partner! I wanted to make that happen, so how?

I'd tried before with some of the usual methods: dating apps, for example. But the first thing I did was delete those. Although I know some great people who got together through these apps and ended up getting married, I didn't feel it was the way that I was going to meet the person I was looking for.

I also didn't focus on dating at all for the first few months after the ayahuasca experience. I'd learned that first I needed to sort myself out a little more, or else I'd end up with the same problems as before. So that's what I did.

As time went by, I was feeling stronger and more stable than I had felt in all my life, and it felt right to start putting more effort in again. I went to a few different activities where I felt I might meet someone I was looking for.

I tried yoga, cultural exchange events, different ceremonies, hiking and so on. To begin with, nothing really came of my efforts. There were a couple of people who I thought I was interested in, but when I went to visit them or got to know them better, it didn't lead to anything.

I also made another major decision – one of the best I have ever made: no more porn! And maybe it goes without saying, but certainly no more prostitutes either!

I'd recently read about the concept of semen retention. This stems from the Eastern philosophy of semen being a man's seed of life, his energy, his aura. The more we waste our seed watching porn, imaging unrealistic scenarios on Instagram and so on, the more we lose our aura and the less attractive we are – to ourselves and to others. It made perfect sense.

It was difficult at first. Porn and masturbation are real addictions, and after so many years, it took a while to break them. I had numerous setbacks along the way.

As I began to gain control over these addictive instincts and the search for instant gratification, my confidence and energy were hugely boosted. I was more sure of who I was and what I was really looking for, and I knew the person I was searching for would feel it too.

There was one woman who had never truly left my mind, but I'd never followed up with her.

I'd been back to Ayahuasca House a few times since my first visit and had some equally tough but equally magical times there. I always got on well with the team: Renato, Sabina, Darsi and the various musicians who passed through. They felt like family, and it was a happy place to be.

I was about to return to Medellin from Villavicencio, where I'd been visiting a friend, Dani, for a few days, when my mind came back to Darsi, the woman I'd considered asking out after my first retreat nine months ago.

An ayahuasca ceremony was due to take place on the Saturday I was travelling back from Bogota. The house was just ten minutes from the airport, so I figured I'd go and have a beautiful ceremony and see why this curiosity in Darsi had suddenly been piqued. A few people I knew from Medellin were also up at the ceremony, and it was a really nice atmosphere from the second I arrived.

It was a tough ceremony. I was going through a lot in wondering what to do, and when I needed support, Darsi was there. I felt in this moment that she was the one, but suddenly all my fears came back.

I knew that now was the time to face up to these fears and act. Not in the middle of the ceremony, but when the moment came the next day.

Reflection 17: Porn

In my opinion, porn is one of the biggest plagues that society is facing. I'm not judging anyone; I watched it from age fourteen to age thirty. But I think we need to start talking about it.

For me, it took me away from the present and put me in a place of imagining others where I thought I wanted to be. I also knew the people taking part probably didn't want to be there.

Instead of being out in the real-world meeting people and forming real connections, I was sitting behind a computer feeling lonely. It drained my energy. It also activates the same instant gratification centres as drugs, bringing short-term pleasure followed by longer-term lows. It's been said to help contribute towards erectile dysfunction too.

It's an addiction that's been well on the rise, but it's not talked about. We need to start discussing the negatives it's bringing people and the positives of leaving it behind: more energy, more connection, higher self-worth, a better hormonal balance, and so much more.

Masturbation has its benefits, such as connecting with ourselves and our bodies. We all have natural instincts after all. But when it comes to porn, even at the level of just looking at an Instagram model, I'm not sure. Where we're going with AI, sex robots and virtual reality sexual experiences is a little terrifying.

More young men are staying at home and isolating themselves than ever before, and porn and everything that comes with it is surely making this worse.

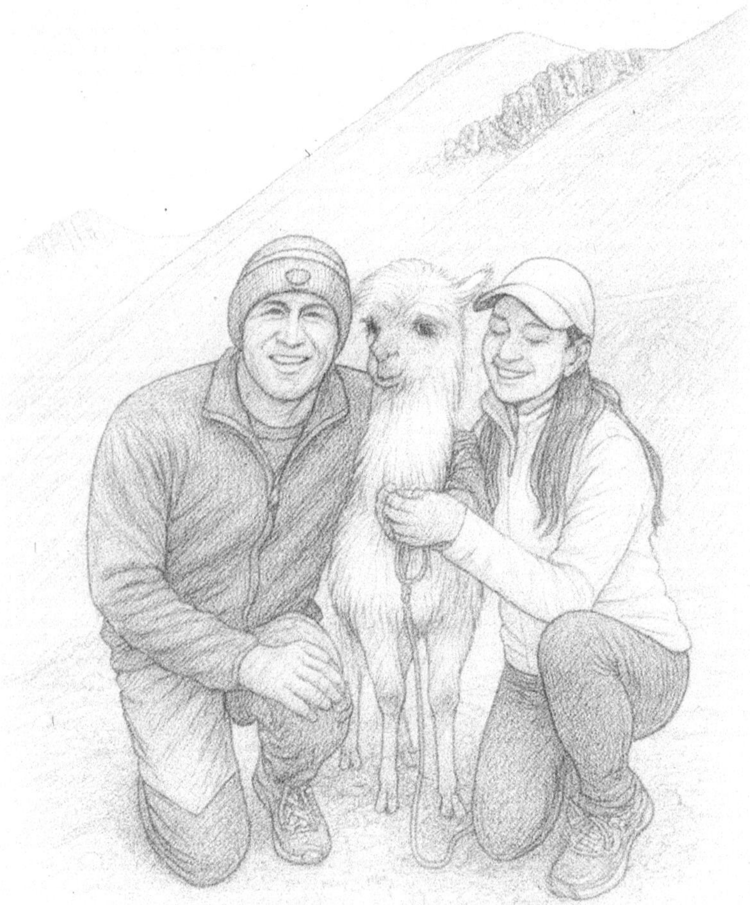

18. The Real One

Darsi has an amazing background.

She grew up in a humble Catholic family of farmers in a part of the Colombian countryside where tomatoes were grown. She lived with her parents, brother and sister in a small house; there was no Wi-Fi, and the cooking was done on a wood-fired stove. The area was also home to a few second homes for people from Medellin, and it turned out that Sabina's mother had a second home very close to Darsi's parents.

Darsi's mum, Adela, occasionally helped Sabina's mum, Sandra, in the garden. One day, when Renato, Sabina and Darsi's family were together at Sandra's house, Sabina noticed something special in Darsi from the look in her eyes when she was just twelve. Darsi had also always dreamed of more than the traditional lifestyle which was what many people followed in those areas. Women would mostly look after the house and cook for their husbands, who worked in the fields.

Out of nothing and thanks to the look in Darsi's eyes that day, Sabina and Renato offered to take her to the capital, Bogota, with them for a month during the school holidays. Darsi's parents agreed: they saw it as a good opportunity for her to do something different.

Darsi loved her time away with them experiencing a completely new life. She'd only been to Medellin once or twice in her life before, spending the rest of the time in the countryside or occasionally in the small village of Guarne, which had only a couple of thousand inhabitants.

It wasn't too long before Darsi was back to the country life again, but she had one more stint in the city – this time in Medellin, with Sabina's sister Valerie. Darsi was sixteen at the time. She went to school there for a few months before returning home to her parents and her small country school. She continued there, working odd farm jobs when she wasn't studying.

When Darsi turned eighteen, she had no idea what to do. She knew what she didn't want, but she had no idea what she *did* want. That's when she called Sabina again. From that moment when Darsi was twelve, there had been a shared love between them. Sabina said Darsi could come and stay with them, and help round the house; they'd just started running the ayahuasca retreats, so she could help get the house organised for that too. And from the age of eighteen to twenty-one – this point in my story – that's what she did.

So, it came to that morning after the ceremony, when I knew I had to act.

Darsi was, still is, and always will be an angel. There's no more accurate way to describe her. She has a heart so caring, an empathy so deep, a beauty far beyond looks, a constant desire to search for more, a mystery, a magic, a way of being that is beyond words. Her love and connection with children is past extraordinary. Anyone who's seen her with children sees this instantly.

I felt all this a little at the first retreat, but that morning I was seeing it in clear letters.

Of course, like all of us, Darsi has her faults, but anyone wanting to start a relationship blindly ignores those. Right then, I just saw hearts and passion.

It came to the moment I'd been working up to. Time to let her know, ask her out. I felt good; I felt free...

But I didn't act. I bottled it, we had a basic conversation and then I left.

Fuck.

Back in my apartment in Envigado, I was wondering why, after everything I'd done to bring myself forward, I couldn't do something so simple for fear of rejection.

It's astounding how this fear holds people back so much in life.

Fear had stopped me on so many occasions in the past, and here it was in my face again. Logically, it's so obvious: if you don't go for it, you've lost anyway, so just take the shot. But taking that shot can be so difficult. The only way to get over that is to just do it.

I wasn't going to let one slip get in the way of the woman of my dreams! I was frustrated, but I was going to make sure we met again as soon as I possibly could, so I could ask her out.

It was only a week before I saw her again and had the chance to take the shot. The fear was still there, but it wasn't going to stop me again!

When I asked Darsi out, I also let her know how I felt. I didn't go over the top, but I told her enough to make it clear. No bullshit, no games. Just a simple conversation.

After ten months of knowing each other, a connection more than just a friendship had begun to form, and I was excited, nervous, happy and terrified about seeing where this could lead.

The next Saturday, we were heading out. I was almost shaking; she was too, I could tell. We went to a popular juice bar, Justo, in Poblado, the tourist area of Medellin. We chilled there for a while, had a walk round the neighbourhood, went for a foot massage afterwards, and followed it up with a pizza. It was fantastic. Everything went perfectly, and Darsi was simply perfect!

This time, I wasn't too little; I wasn't not good enough. I knew I was perfect for her too. We were perfect, and I'd finally found what for thirty-one years of my life I'd been looking for and wanting more than ever. It had been a long and painful road to get here, with heartbreaks and upsets along the way. But now I simply knew. I was more sure of this than anything else in my life.

People often comment on how lucky we are to have found each other. But I assure you, there's no luck in it. There never is with these things.

From the first date onwards, things proceeded with the same love, passion and happiness they had begun with.

We've certainly had our fair share of challenges, difficulties and arguments – many bigger than I'd had with anyone else before. But all the lessons I'd learned have served to turn these into tipping points where our love and connection grows stronger and deeper.

She's the perfect woman for me. She's the woman I'll have children with,* and the woman I'll spend the rest of my life with. Of that I've never been surer of anything. Even in our hardest moments.

Some people give up too early on relationships, or they're not truly right. But with Darsi, I know that can never happen.

My proposal, and our marriage, were something to remember for decades. More romantic than I and she could have ever imagined!

I've never been one for needing a ring and a piece of paper from the church or the government to show my love, and neither has Darsi. I'd never really liked weddings either. Especially in the UK, where they often turn into people getting smashed at a party with loud music at

* One day...

the end. After all, drunk people are very annoying. I have experience: I was one for many years!

Here's the story: I'd initially had a visa in Colombia through setting up a business, but this 'business' didn't do much other than get me a visa. When I needed to renew my visa and the 'business' didn't have much real activity to show for itself, it wasn't going to be possible to renew it this way. That put me in an awkward spot.

How to solve it?

Marriage.

I proposed to Darsi on my sofa, explaining my visa situation and the solution of marriage.

Romance was somewhat missing.

She was chilled about it, and a month or so later, after gathering all the papers together, we got married in a government office in the village of Guarne. This office was just a room in a house, where random people were walking around serving admin needs. The 'ceremony' took about twenty minutes, we were dressed in clothes that we wore every day, and when we left, we celebrated with a croissant nearby before heading back to our normal lives. To be fair, this probably was my dream wedding. I genuinely don't like weddings.

If any Colombian authorities are reading, we're more in love than ever, we're very happy making Colombia a better place, and this marriage is truer and more genuine than words can possibly describe, even if the ceremony and proposal don't reflect that. Please don't revoke my visa.

Darsi and I weren't living together at this point, but shortly after the wedding we moved into a little wooden cabin with a beautiful garden out in the Colombian countryside, where we still are today. We love it here.

My parents didn't know we were married until we saw them about six months later. They'd never met Darsi.** The first night we saw them, I told them. My mum began to cry in happiness, my dad said he knew I'd always do something like this, and that was that.

They get on amazingly. Most importantly for my parents, they're so happy I found such a truly beautiful woman in every sense of the word.

One other thing to touch on: since the first ayahuasca retreat and turning my head towards natural ways of healing, I was determined to never touch Viagra or Cialis ever again. I talked through all my past problems with Darsi. Though things weren't always perfect to begin with and the nerves certainly kicked in from time to time, it didn't take long until the issue was fully resolved through a combination of honesty, trust, and an all-round better way of living life.

When there's nothing to hide, the fear subsides, and when there's real connection, the true intimacy can take over.

** Apart from on a couple of video calls.

Overcoming this issue felt like another miracle. It was a painful, embarrassing and emasculating issue, but it was one that I now know is common for a large number of people. If that's you, it's fine; it happens, there is hope, and there's a natural, healthy and real solution away from the pills. If I can do it, so can you.

It would also be wrong not to mention Brett, a guy who I'd met at this stage in my life, who helped me step into this problem head on, take it in my stride, step into my sexual power, and move closer to becoming the man I knew I truly was, but at times had left behind because of fear and self-doubt.

I'm so thankful that I only truly discovered this sexual power at this point, with this angel. Everything happens for a reason; I could now see it clearly. If I'd had sexual confidence in my younger days, I'd have made a mess of everything: women, partners and everything else.

All the lessons I'd learned before were important for reaching where I am today. They might not have made sense at the time, but now it's clear as day.

Sex in its purest form is a celebration of life, intimacy and love, and that's what I am now able to experience with the purest angel on this planet.

Reflection 18: Magical

Real love!

It's the most beautiful thing I've experienced. It's what I'd always wanted, and it took me so long to find it, but to be with Darsi made every day of waiting worth it.

I'm sure these feelings are only amplified by a million when kids come along too.

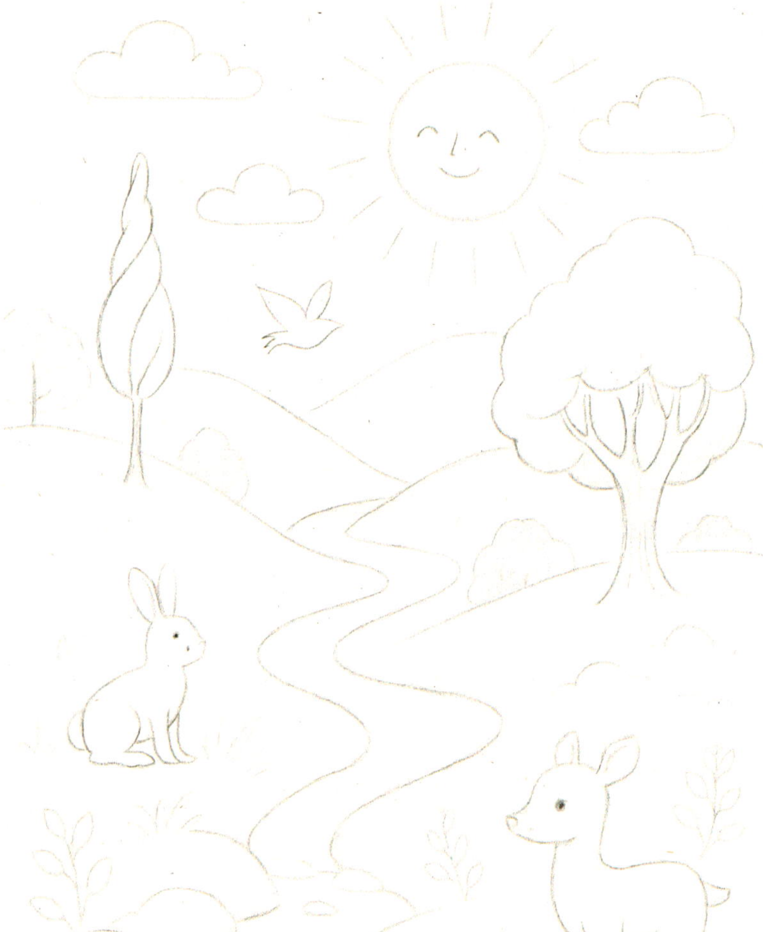

19. Kids and the World

I never wanted kids.

I used to think that if I ever did want kids, I'd adopt but never have my own. When I was too messed up, I saw the world as too messed up as well, and I didn't want to bring a kid into this place. And it's easy to see the world as messed up, with everything we read in the papers and see on the news.

I was that convinced that I almost had a vasectomy shortly before the ayahuasca retreat in 2019. Shout out to my oldest friend and current urologist James, who talked me out of that one. I'm not sure if I'd have gone through with it, but his words certainly made sure I didn't try

As I changed the way I saw myself, the way I saw the world also changed, and vice versa. The world is a truly beautiful and magical place, filled with thousands of random acts of kindness and love from millions of people every day.

Of course, many truly awful things happen too. But my view is that our society, the mainstream agenda and our minds are configured to steer us towards looking for the negatives rather than the positives.

I don't have a delusional mindset around positivity: it's important to be aware of the shit that's going on in the world. That way, if possible, we can take action to try and improve what's going on.

But if you're in a situation where you're able to read this book, it's likely you have the good fortune not to be living in a zone of pure war and destruction, for example. If you look around you today, you'll see people trying to make the best of their lives, smiling, helping other people, making mistakes and learning. You'll see beautiful trees, changing weather, children playing, dogs running and dreams happening – and it's magical.

Often, we simply spend too much time focusing on the negatives to see this. Unless we're going to do something to change those negatives, this saps our energy and vibration away, leaving us with less of that to genuinely help others. The magic that happens around us every day passes us by.

I now appreciate this magic every day,* and it's a joy to be alive. I know how fortunate I am to have been dealt the cards I have, and the best way to celebrate that fortune is to play them as best as I can and try to make a difference where I can.

The way I now see it, the best way to celebrate what Darsi and I have together, in this magical world, is to bring one or two more little people into it!

---

* Or at least on most days...

Reflection 19: The Most Beautiful Thing I Can Imagine

A family!

It's the most beautiful thing I can imagine.

And I'm sure I won't have to imagine it for too much longer.

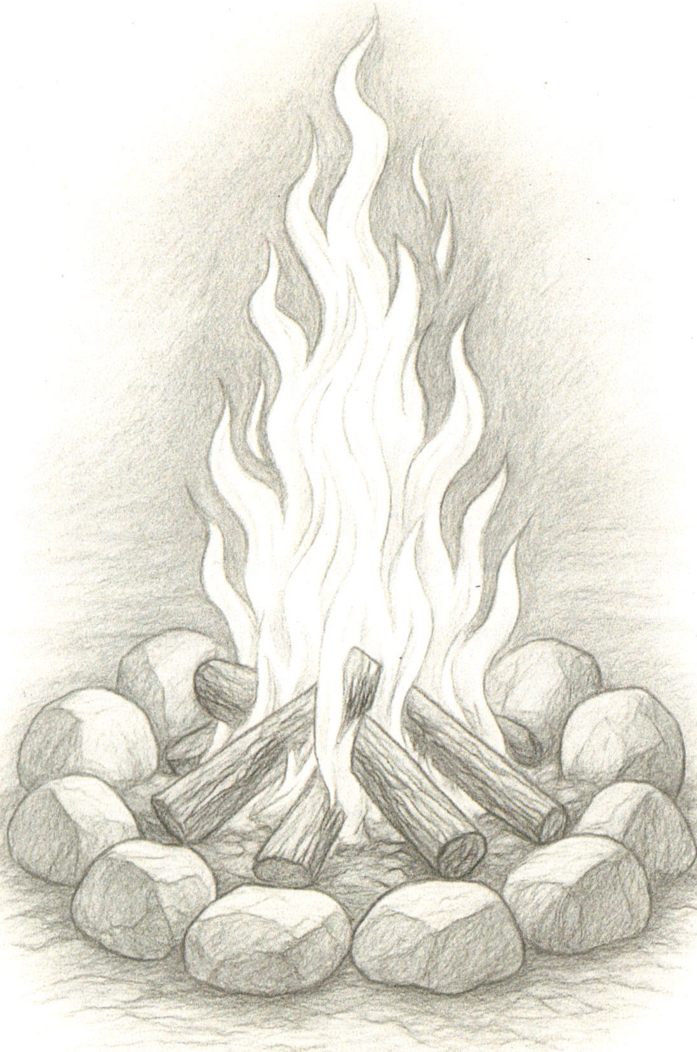

20. A Shaman?

Now I'm married, I'm working in a decent job with Mikey, I have good people round me in Colombia, and my health and wellbeing are better than ever. What more could I want?

Since my first ayahuasca retreat, my vision has been to learn more about ayahuasca and eventually to bring it to the UK.

To be able to serve ayahuasca responsibly takes a lot of time, presence, and discipline. It's not something you take once, buy off the street and bring with you to give to anyone. Even so, unfortunately that does happen in some cases, and it can be dangerous.

It's such a powerful substance, and some very intense things can happen during ceremonies. It's important to take time to learn from experts on how to manage these things, and I continue to observe and learn.

I'm learning from Renato and his guide, Taita Don Gerardo, who descends from the Llanacona indigenous tribe in Colombia. His grandfather was a master shaman, and now Don Gerardo is taking the tradition forward with love.

As I write this I'm at his home – on a beautiful piece of land to the North of Putumayo in Colombia, during a week-long retreat with a few other people I'm close to: Bennet, Gokula, Renato, Sabina, two Austrian herbologists (Mikaela and Reiner), and Josh (a British guy I've just met).

It's my second time here. The first time, we cooked ayahuasca. This is an incredibly intensive process. First, it involves preparing the ayahuasca vine and the chakruna leaf, the two ingredients in ayahuasca. They are then cooked over a fire for anything from thirty-six to seventy-two hours. It's important to remain present during the process to make sure it all goes right. It's hard work.

I was cooking ayahuasca under Don Gerardo's guidance with the help of his friend, Don Aureliano. These two people have an incredible amount of wisdom that I was able to observe, feel and learn from.

One of the challenges in my longer-term vision of bringing ayahuasca to England is that in the UK and in many other parts of the world, ayahuasca* remains a class A drug, considered to be on the same level as heroin or cocaine. The same classification has been given to many other psychedelics too. This seems simply absurd, because when they are worked with responsibly, these plants have the power to transform and heal people's lives.

Psychedelics I believe do need some form of regulation. If they're not used in the right way or environment, or the people serving them don't have the proper

* More specifically, the psychedelic component it contains: DMT.

knowledge, experience, permission and care, they can be dangerous.

But to simply deny their use to so many people who could benefit from them is sad. After all, if alcohol – a drug that leads to more deaths than any other substance – is legal, then why aren't other natural substances that have a genuine healing effect?

I know psychedelics and ayahuasca aren't for everyone. My dad came to a retreat and certainly didn't have the most beautiful experience. I believe this was mainly because he was coming to see what I was so passionate about, rather than for his own personal reasons. For the magic to happen, you have to really want to look inside yourself.

What he did get was to see his son in an environment that he cared about, that was helping a lot of people, and that made him happy. After all, what more can a father want than that?

My mum is a little more conservative in her views on psychedelics. However, she now feels similar to my dad, even if she finds it harder to relate to and understand.

I remain hopeful that scientific research, shared experiences and the shifts in the wider political environment will make ayahuasca and other psychedelics more available to people. It will take time, but I have a long time to live and much more to learn. I'm happy to wait. It's also my hope that the true, responsible indigenous cultures and guardians, rather than the pharmaceutical industry, can lead the way on this journey.

Many people do work with ayahuasca in the UK and in other parts of the world where it's illegal, but I'm not going to take that risk. I have a wife and an incredible life here in Colombia, and I don't want to do anything that could spoil that.

Another difficulty in achieving my vision is that I've felt a little disconnected from ayahuasca and my learnings in the last few months. To become a shaman, you need real presence and commitment – and I've lost those recently.

This could be because I realise that ayahuasca isn't for everyone. It's not the only medicine, technique or practice that can transform lives; there are many different paths. I also see too many people taking ayahuasca regularly but making no positive changes.

Life moves in different ways, and right now my focus is elsewhere.

Maybe my full presence and commitment to this vision will return one day; maybe it won't. But I do still see ayahuasca as the most powerful tonic for life that there is.

I'm a little biased, but who can blame me? It helped to transform my life!

Reflection 20: If You Feel the Call

It would be magical if these medicines, which can have such a positive and healing effect on so many people, became more mainstream and legal, and were managed in a responsible way across the world.

The good news is that they already are in countries like Brazil, Colombia and Peru.

If you find yourself being called towards ayahuasca, there are many incredible shamans who could open the space for you to walk into. If you're willing and open, it could help change your life. Just do your research first and find a good, safe and responsible place.

If not, there are so many different paths. I hope you're already on yours, or if not, that you find it soon.

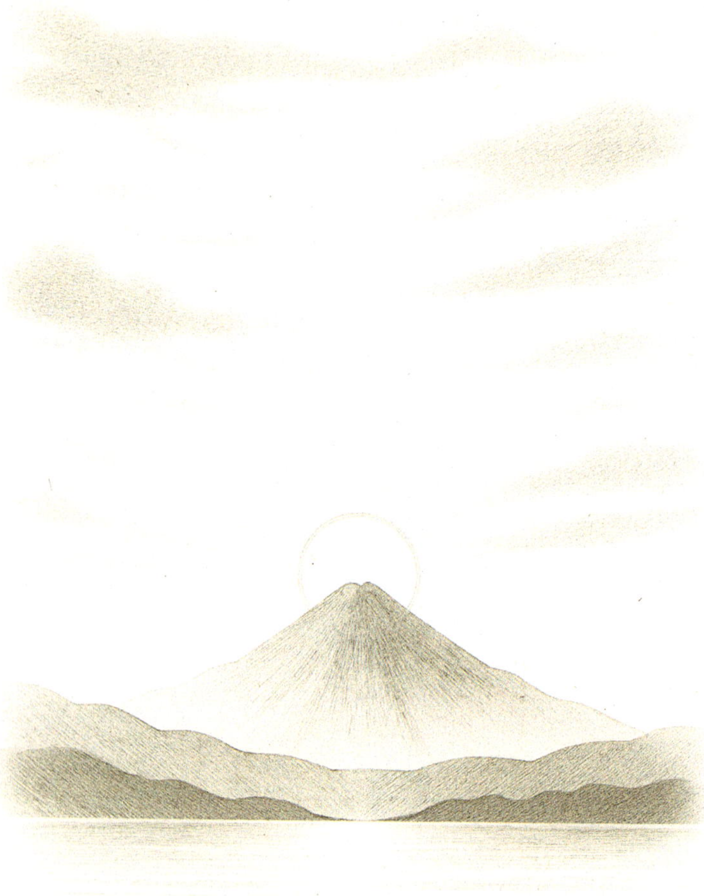

21. Sexual Power

As I've continued to move forward and grow with time, I've developed the inner confidence and presence to talk to any woman. I'm no longer too intimidated to start a conversation with a woman I find attractive.

I used to not even be able to look a woman in the eye, let alone talk to her or get together with her. Now here I am, feeling as if I could get together with almost anyone. This is a power I'd only ever dreamed of having, and one that I was so envious of when I saw it in others.

Here's the catch: I don't want it. I have zero interest.

Ironically, that's where some of the power comes from.

Sure, I'm like any other testosterone-filled male, with urges that come here and there. But I just tell them I'm not interested. I live in my own world, show no interest, and keep being my own weird self.

If ever I get talking to someone and I feel the slightest tinge of sexual energy, I drop in that I'm married within about two seconds, even if it has no relation to what we're talking about. The energy ends in that moment, and I can move forwards with true love, knowing there'll only ever be one girl I want to be with.

Reflection 21: 'God Has a Funny Sense of Humour'

When I talked with Mikey about this, the way he put it made me laugh. We've both lacked confidence around women in the past. He too now has a sexual confidence that he'd never thought possible, but he has a true angel of a wife who he'd do anything for.

He said: 'God has a funny sense of humour. We think we really want something for so much of our lives, then when we can have it, we don't want it.'

Some people let the temptation win. It's not worth it.

Family and love. They beat everything.

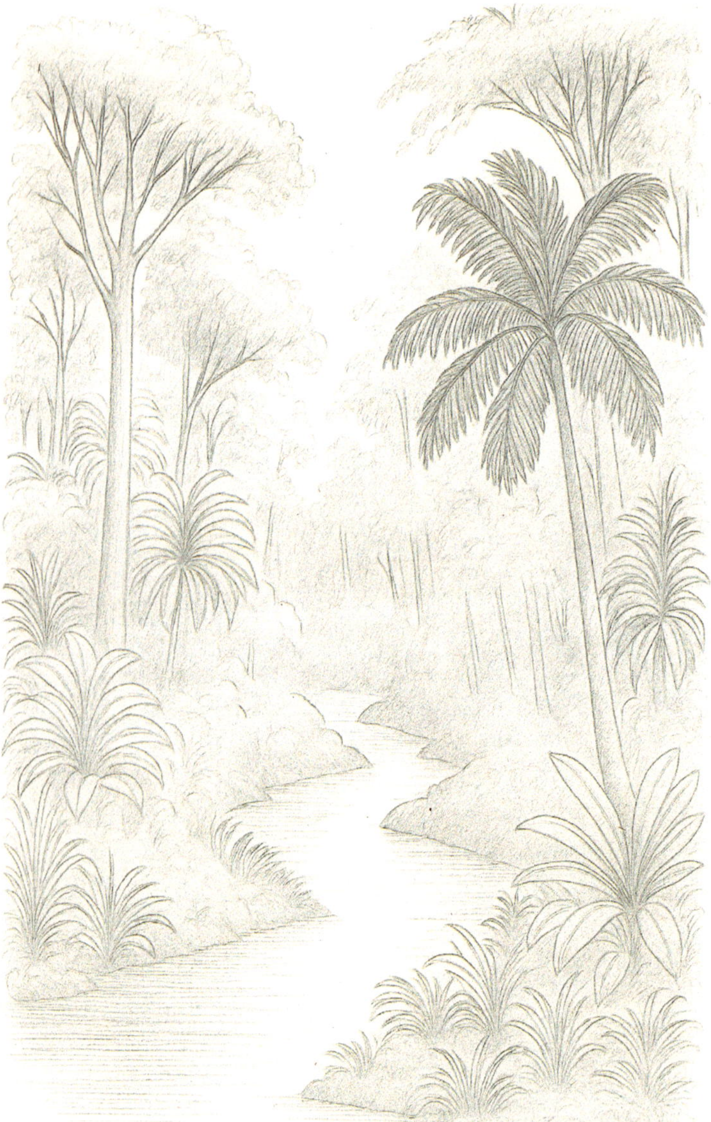

22. Creating Paradise

Another dream began to manifest from nothing.

Renato and I were talking one day around this time, and he's like me. Always searching for something more. After one ayahuasca ceremony, completely *chumando*,* we decided we wanted *much* more, and we began looking for land.

The world was in a bit of a crazy place, and we're slightly crazy people.

We weren't looking for a small section of land in the city, but a larger piece of nature further afield. In Colombia, land in or around the big cities is now very expensive too, but out in the countryside it's more reasonable.

We also wanted to create something a little different. We didn't really know what we were looking for, but we wanted somewhere we'd be able to grow food organically and protect nature. Given the continuing decrease in the quality of supermarket food – from pesticide-sprayed vegetables to highly injected meats and ultra-processed whatever else – we wanted to grow our own food, and

* The spiritual word for 'high'.

have our own water supply.** We also wanted to plant trees – as many as our piece of land would allow.

Initially we went looking for somewhere to create our paradise in San Rafael, a beautiful village on the tourist trail about three hours from Medellin. But there were two major problems. Firstly, most of the rainforest and other trees there had been cut down to make way for farming, development or tourism, which wasn't what we were looking for. Secondly, it's a popular place so land there costs quite a lot of money. However, in our search we met a man called Don Pedro, who informed us that he had over 300 hectares*** of land for sale in Argelia.

We had absolutely no idea where Argelia was. Nor does half of Colombia. It's a tiny village in the middle of nowhere. It's an hour past another village, Sonson, which is an hour and a half after another village, La Union, which is another hour and a half from Medellin. All these villages are well off the tourist trail. Unless you're from there, there's no real reason to go.

At first, we had no interest in this land, it was simply too far away, but Pedro had shown us some photos, and it looked magical. As Renato and I were talking, we thought, 'Why don't we just go and visit it?' This involved planning a three-day trip with Pedro. After all, the land wasn't actually in Argelia, but one hour past the village down a dirt track in a 4x4 and then a further hour's hike down

** With no fluoride.

*** 740 acres.

a steep muddy track. I'm fairly sure I was the first British person to visit Argelia, but I'm certain I was the first British person to visit where we were going.

It really was in the middle of nowhere. Even I wasn't prepared for how far it was. But it was more magical than the photos portrayed. It had a river running through the whole property, 200 hectares of untouched rainforest and 100 hectares of farmland or field where we could grow things or build, and twenty-five further water sources. In the valley around it there were twenty-six families of rural farmers, mostly growing coffee or farming cows. This friendly community worked together to support each other. It all had a nice vibe.

We fell in love. We didn't really think. The whole thing made no sense, but we figured that maybe we could create a new community – a 'mini country' – on this land.

We tried not to show too much interest so as not to weaken our negotiating position if we decided to go ahead, but we also kept referring to everything as 'ours' from the first moment.

Two weeks later we were back – me with Darsi, and Renato with Sabina – to see what they all thought of it. It was impossible not to be amazed by the beauty of the place, but they were less keen on the location.

Still, we all concluded, mainly with Renato and my enthusiasm, why not? And a couple of months later we were the owners of 300 hectares of land. We left it as it was for a few months while we planned what to do. We then went down to look at it with a friend of ours, Jeronimo, and his family, who have a community of their own. They advised us on a few things to do.

There was plentiful wood in the area for construction. We didn't touch any healthy or growing trees, only the ones that were dying or old: we were there to preserve the beauty in the area. There was plenty of sand and rock, but not much else. Everything else needed to be brought from the village or further afield. This meant sending it on the *escaleras*, the large trucks that people used for transport round there, to the point at the top of the valley, and then organising for it all to be brought down the final hour's trek by mule. All the wood we cut, the sand we collected and everything we'd brought in had to be taken to the construction point by mule too.

We had a good team of locals who helped us get most of it done, although we did get involved where we could. There were so many logistics to organise and so many things went wrong, but we learned a lot too and it was fun!

And a year and a half later, we had our first social space built which could also be used in future for ceremonies if we wanted, with twelve very small Japanese-style wooden pod rooms beneath it. We also built a beautiful wooden house for Alvaro, the *mayordomo*,**** and his wife and two children to live. Things were taking shape.

**** Land Steward.

We also began planting. With this, we had no idea what we were doing. We had a clear vision: growing completely organic and self-sustaining food on part of the land, and reforesting the rest of it with native trees. We initially brought in 2,700 trees, a full truckload. That's a lot! They were tiny trees, but still, we were soon to learn that it's a lot of work to get them in the ground.

Most of the cost of planting these trees is not in the tree itself but preparing the land, digging the holes, getting the natural fertiliser, and bringing the trees down to the land by mule. It took us almost three months to get them all in the ground.

We were also complete amateurs who thought planting a tree was as simple as making a hole and putting a bit of natural fertiliser down. As it turns out, in such infertile soil that has been used as a cow field for years, where nothing grows but weeds and ferns, it takes so much more work than this. More than two years on, we're still trying to get better at planting and trying to make up for our initial ignorance to ensure the trees grow.

We've learned a lot. We need to fertilise the soil with a range of different nutrients, found in a combination of natural substances (mainly chicken manure, but much more besides). We need to ensure the weeds and ferns don't consume the trees. We need to keep the leaf-eating ants away. It's taken a huge amount of energy and resources, but most of the trees are now thriving and some are over 10 metres tall.

We approached the food in a similar way at first, planting fruit trees and other things with just a little basic fertiliser until we realised that they needed much more than this. This is the point where I invited a guy I knew, Daniel, who did organic farming, to help us out. He basically criticised[*****] all the strategies we'd used. We had to make better fertiliser, diversify what we planted to add nutrients and organic matter to the soil, keep the weeds away in a more natural and efficient way, and more.

Daniel was a great help until one day he messaged me to say he could no longer assist us. I wondered why: had we done something wrong? It turned out that he had become very religious, and working with people who were involved with ayahuasca and psychedelics didn't align with his values. Still, we were very grateful to him for his help and I'm still in touch with him today.

He put us in touch with two real experts in regenerative farming, Felipe and Melisa, from a company called Bioma, who are now supporting us with everything. We've since planted another 2,500 trees and many more seeds in a self-sustaining way, and our rainforest is beginning to appear. This part of the dream is turning into a reality.

The vision to create a community there has been a different story for two main reasons. The first is obvious: money.

***** With love.

The project was costing a huge amount to develop, and our finances to keep supporting it were running thin. None of us ever lived there full time, as we were focused on our bread-and-butter projects and living nearer to Medellin, but we were visiting a couple of times a month to manage everything.

The second issue is something that affects many regions across Colombia. The region became more politically unstable, and there were new and growing risks, with various military and guerilla groups active in the wider region.

We've only ever had good relationships with the people in the area, and we've never seen or experienced any trouble, and we know that will continue. But still, it makes you think.

Given that we were so low on resources as well, we decided to pause our community vision for the time being.

We still visit a lot. It's an amazing place and it's a project that we'll always enjoy. We'll continue to expand it gradually.

More importantly, in the meantime, we'll continue to plant as many trees as we can and protect as much rainforest as possible. The project is truly beautiful, and you can see it on our YouTube channel at 'Yacumadre'.

Our ultimate dream is to create the largest natural reserve in Colombia. To achieve this is going to require a huge amount of support. Our not-for-profit organisation has received some support and funding, but we're many millions away from the goal.

Even so, we've come a long way: more than 5,000 trees in the ground, 200 hectares of virgin rainforest protected, and twenty-five water sources beginning to flourish again – and we haven't even begun.

Now, at the end of 2025, we're putting a further 3,900 trees in the ground too!

Reflection 22: A Vision Bigger than Myself

Why not dream?

I now have a goal bigger than myself to keep me entertained and focused, and that's to create the largest natural reserve in Colombia.

The project is a lot of work, but it's a lot of fun and it keeps me grounded and focused.

Learning and understanding how to plant in harmony with nature is also something I love.

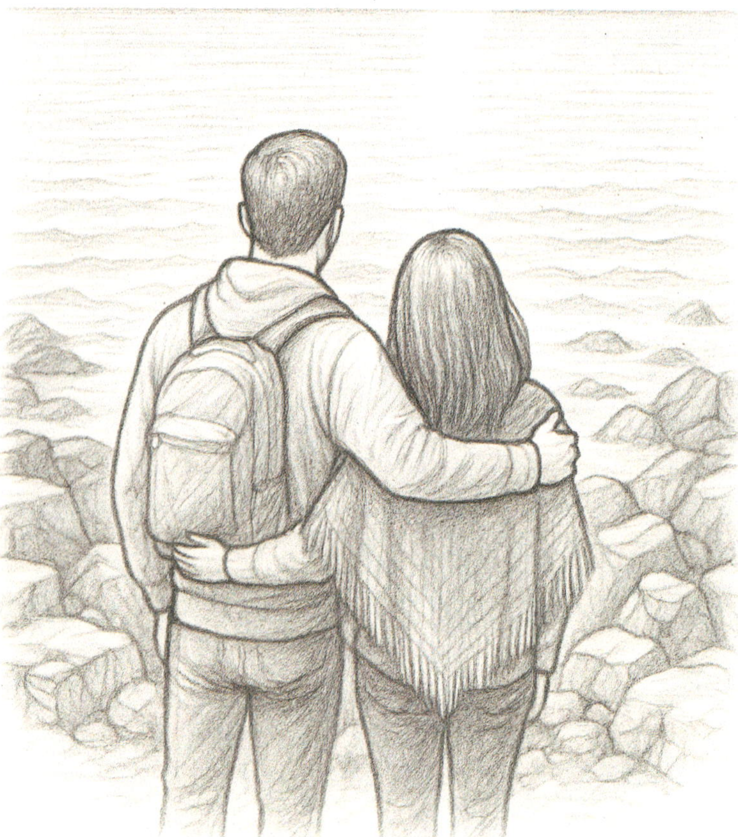

23. Now and Next

That brings me to today. I'm still working with Mikey, part time, in my sales role. I'm still very involved with ancestral medicines and ayahuasca, albeit with a little less focus. I'm more in love with Darsi than I've ever been. I'm still working towards creating the largest natural reserve in Colombia.

I'm still always searching for what's next, pushing boundaries, messing up, learning, and moving forwards. And I'm still taking things to extremes.

I've now got an ice bath behind my cabin set at 3.5 degrees, which until recently I was hopping into every morning. I trained solidly in jiu-jitsu for a year, entering a competition in which I lost in the first round. I've been going to the gym three or four times a week and I've gained 4 kg of muscle – something I've never done before.

I'm beginning to learn that taking things to extremes isn't the way.

I'd have rather discovered this by doing it than by not pushing myself to my limits, and I have no regrets about that. But I recently started doing the human biography therapy I'd been introduced to by Sabina at Ayahuasca House, looking deeper into my personality and how I live my life. It's showing me how I can continue to grow and step further into my potential and purpose.

And the extremes are something I've been contemplating. Yanina, with whom I do the therapy, shows my 'personality' as a pendulum between a monk and a monster. I think that's right: swinging between extremes and often losing sight of the middle ground.

I'm finally taking that lesson on board. I've stopped hopping in the ice bath as much. I've moved away from jiu-jitsu to more casual boxing. And I'm trying to take a slightly slower and calmer approach to life.

It's working. I'm enjoying life more. I know who I am. I stand up straight. I smile. I laugh. I cry. I have faith.

We'll see what happens next.

The depths I went to with my personal demons in my earlier life may be surprising to some; and some may think the transformation I experienced later on is nothing more than bullshit and drugs.

Maybe they're right.

You can make up your mind.

I've made up mine.

9781908770943

SD - #0080 - 020226 - C0 - 203/127/11 - PB - 9781908770943 - Matt Lamination